COPYRIGHT 2012 L HARHARI SINGH
THE DIVINE PORTAL

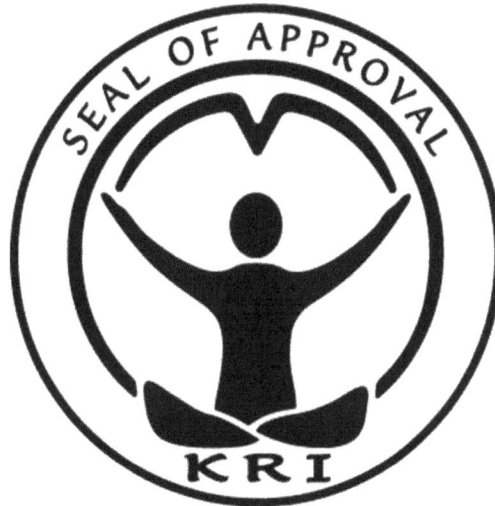

MANTRALOGY:
AN ANTHOLOGY OF SACRED CHANTS

MANTRAS USED IN KUNDALINI YOGA AS TAUGHT BY YOGI BHAJAN®

This compilation is dedicated to the transformation & evolution of the Entire world's population of Hue-Mans, Being

Anthos = Flower
Logos = To gather or collect

TABLE OF CONTENTS

Compiled & Transliterated by L HarHari Singh
From & Inspired by the Teachings of Yogi Bhajan

WWW.THEDIVINEPORTAL.COM

♥ The words "Kundalini Yoga" hereby refer to Kundalini Yoga As Taught By Yogi Bhajan®

ACKNOWLEDGEMENTS

This manual is the product of great inspiration and love from many beings. By the Grace of God, as well as the assistance from many, this Anthology has become possible.

Thank you, Yogi Bhajan for carrying these teachings to the West. Thank you Gurmukh Kaur & Gurushabd Singh for having been my teachers and allowing me to have known you, serve with you and learn from you. Thank you, Gurudass Kaur, for being an amazing inspiration and for sharing your musical gifts. Thank you, Guru Singh, for your mastery of words and your wisdom. Thank you Sada Sat Kaur Khalsa. Thank you, Snatam Kaur Khalsa for sharing your angelic voice and presence and for bringing the Shabd Guru to so many ears and hearts around the world. Thank you, Guru Ganesha Singh for your guitar riffs and wild stories about Woodstock. Thank you, Sat Purkh Kaur Khalsa, for letting me crash on your friends couch that year we met at Solstice (and for your divine music too!). Thank you Mirabai Ceiba, Sat Kirin Kaur, Hari Bhajan Kaur, Guru Raj Kaur, Gurunam, Niranjan Kaur, Sat Kartar Kaur, Singh Kaur, Siri Dharma Kaur, Simran Kaur, Gurudass Singh, Harjinder Singh Gil, Sangeet Kaur, Gurucharan Singh, Carioca, Bachan Kaur, Aurora, Alka Yagnik, Sada Sat Singh, Sat Nam Singh, Ram Singh, Pritpal Kaur, Wah!, Sat Jivan Singh & Sat Jivan Kaur, Shaina Noll, Bhai Joginder Singh Riaar and to all those unnamed who have blessed us with sacred music in the Kundalini Yoga tradition.

A very special thank you to Singh Brothers Publishing (www.singhbrothers.com) for granting me permission to reproduce translation excerpts from Sacred Nitnem. Very special thank you to Sant Singh Khalsa, Md. for permission to reprint your beautiful translations. Thank you Spirit Voyage Music (www.spiritvoyage.com) for providing supplemental assistance for translations. Thank you Gurumustuk Singh Khalsa, a.k.a. Mr Sikhnet (www.mrsikhnet.com) for finding me translations to the 2 words I could not find a translation for anywhere else. You are a gem, Dear Brother. Thank you Snatam Kaur Khalsa, Sopurkh Singh Khalsa and their wonderful web team at www.snatamkaur.com for translation assistance.

Thank you www.rajkaregakhalsa.net for additional translation support. Thank you to the Kundalini Research Institute-KRI (www.kriteachings.org) for the preservation and promotion of Kundalini Yoga. Thank you to 3HO for the innumerable services you provide for the community. Thank you to Karam Jot Singh, M.A. who I met after one of my workshops at the Midwest Yoga Conference that taught me about the complex relationship between Gurmukhi and Punjabi. Thank you Siri Neel Kaur Khalsa for guiding me through the process of making this manual what it is. Thank you to my parents and to Jennifer "Durga" Ayala-Lawson, my beloved wife, for editing all of the English sections of this manual and for supporting me and my vision to compile this work. Thank you to everyone who was scared to try something new and did it anyway. You inspire me! Thank you. Thank you. Thank you.

Sincerely,
L HarHari Singh
www.TheDivinePortal.com

PRONUNCIATION KEY

The mantras contained within this manual have been transliterated in the most basic system of phonics possible. Each letter will represent a sound that will appear universally throughout the book. In other words, every like letter will represent the same sound every time it appears. The native English speaker may find a need to adjust to habits in pronunciation. Please carefully analyze the table provided below as you begin to adjust your mind to a purely phonetic way of reading words. Remember, as the sound appears once, it will appear throughout. There are virtually no exceptions. If you are familiar with reading any phonetic language, such as Spanish or Hawaiian, you may more easily embrace this system. Otherwise, please take some time to familiarize yourself with the key below:

Symbol	= Read As	In English	Examples (Eng. Pronunciation)
ï	= Ih	as in Win, Fin	*Tïs, Kïn* or *Prïtam* (pri-tum)
i	= Eee	as in Chi	*Bi, Ki* (Kee); *Sïri* (si-ree); *Tis* (Teece)
a, Aa	= Aah	as in Wand, Father*	*Akal, Sat* or *Tribavan* (Tree-bah-vun)
u, ū	= Ooh	as in Tune, True^	*Gūn*, or *Mūkandey* (Moo-kun-day)
e	= Eh	as in Gem, Bell	*Mera, Mela* or *Nehechal* (Ne-he-chal)
o	= Oh	as in Home, Comb, Go	*Choj, Soch* or *Gobïnda* (Go-bin-da)
e+y = ey	= Ay	as in Grey, Prey	*Jey, Hey, Keyra* or *Sagaley* (Sa-ga-lay)
a+i = ai	= I	as in Pry, Aye	*Ajai, Alai, Kai* or *Gavai* (Ga-vie)
a+e = ae	= Eh + Ah	No words in English	*Hae*
h	= h	as in How+	*Wahe, Sahib*, or *Abhai* (Aab-high)

*a & Aa are pronounced identically. Words that begin with 'A' in English tend to take on a harsh 'A' sound (as in 'Ant' or 'Asteroid') or a long 'AY' sound (as in 'Wane' or 'Pail'. The letter 'A' will never represent those sounds in this manual. Words that begin with the 'A' sound are sometimes transliterated with Aa to remind the native English speaker that nothing but a **soft** 'A', as in 'Wash', & the other examples above, is spoken.
Therefore, *Akamey* is pronounced (Ah-ka-may); *Aad* (Ahd or Odd); Nad (Naad or Nod)

^ u & ū are pronounced identically. To overcome the conditioning of the mind, the symbol ū was placed where a native English speaker would be inclined to say *'sun'* rather than *'soon'* when reading the transliteration *Sūn*. 'U' will always be pronounced as a long 'U' or *'oo'* sound.
Therefore, *Mūn* (Moon)

+h is always enunciated; it is never silent. Often it is pronounced as an aspirant sound, meaning, it is not spoken as harshly has a normal 'H' in English. Rather, it has more of a 'breathy' quality. 'H' in combination with the consonants 'S', as "Shoot", and 'C' as in "Chill" are pronounced the same way in this manual.

The sound of r is created by flicking the tongue to the roof of the mouth, about ½" behind the front teeth, similar to Spanish, but further back. This is a very important component to pronouncing mantras in sacred languages. The closest comparison in English would be like pronouncing a D, yet not as hard. To enunciate the r, one must tap the tongue, rather than press it, upward.

All other letters will be pronounced as in English. Some sounds do not transliterate perfectly.

ONG NAMO GURU DEYV NAMO
Adi Mantra - I bow to the Divine Wisdom & Divine Teacher that is within My Self

Ong = Infinite creative energy in manifestation
Namo = Salutations; I bow
Guru = Teacher, wisdom   (Gu = darkness, stickiness; Ru = remover of)
Deyv = That which is divine
Namo = 'Bowing' yet again, sealing in this Power with humility

This mantra is called **The Adi Mantra**. It tunes us in with the Masters of this sacred lineage (Golden Chain) of Kundalini Yoga as Taught by Yogi Bhajan® while connecting with our own divine essence. "**Adi** means first or primal."[1]

How to recite the Adi Mantra
Sit in Easy Pose with you hands pressed together at the center of your chest in Prayer Mudra (Anjali [*Anyali*] Mudra). Press the joints of the thumbs into the sternum. Close your eyes and focus at your third eye point. Inhale deeply and chant the mantra all in one breath. (If your breath is not capable of this, then take a small sip of air after "Ong namo" and then chant the rest of the mantra, extending the sound along as possible. The sound "deyv" is chanted a minor third higher than the other sounds of the mantra. Please see fig. 1[2] below)

Ong . . . .   Namo . . . .   Gu-ru Deyv . . . .   Na - Mo . . . .

Chant this mantra 3-5 times before beginning your Kundalini Yoga practice.

SAT NAM
Truth is My Identity

Sat = Truth   **Nam** = Identity, Name

This affirms our true essence of oneness with all of creation.

When broken down into its primal sound forms it is known as **The Panj Shabd**: SA TA NA MA (*Kirtan Kriya*[3] *Mantra*).

Sa = Infinity, cosmos, beginning   **Na** = Death, change, transformation
Ta = Life, existence   **Ma** = Rebirth

This mantra also embodies the essence of the Hindu Trinity: Brahma, Vishnu & Shiva. **Sa, Ta, Na & Ma** contain the five (*panj*) sounds of the mantra for Kirtan Kriya[4], as well as dozens of other meditations and kriyas. The 5 sounds are 'Sss', 'T', 'Nnn', 'Mmm' & 'Aaa'.

AAD GUREY NAMEH
Mangalacharn Mantra

Aad Gurey Nameh	= I bow to the primal wisdom
Jūgad Gurey Nameh	= I bow to the wisdom true through the ages
Sat Gurey Nameh	= I bow to the true wisdom
Sïri Guru Deyv-ey Nameh	= I bow to the great unseen wisdom

"This is a mantra which clears the clouds of doubt and opens us to guidance and protection. It surrounds the electro-magnetic field with protective light."[5]

Mangalam = Auspicious
Charn = Feet

"This mantra is a way for one to move forward after a difficult or challenging situation."[6]

LONG TIME SUN

May The Long Time Sun Shine Upon You
All Love Surround You
And The Pure Light Within You
Guide Your Way On[7]

This is the closing prayer for Kundalini Yoga classes. The prayer is a line from a song by the *Incredible String Band* that Yogi Bhajan heard as he entered to teach a class in Los Angeles in the early years. It is said that he heard the people gathered for class singing it and he loved it so much, it became the farewell blessing for Kundalini Yoga classes.

AQUARIAN SADHANA MANTRAS 8

Yogi Bhajan gave the following sequence of mantras on June 21, 1992, with instructions to continue using them for morning Sadhana in the following order for 21 years. So, until the year 2013, we are set with the best Sadhana tools possible.

EK ONG KAR ~ *Morning Call - Long Ek Ong Kar (7 minutes)*

Ek Ong Kar Sat Nam Sïri Wahe Guru

There is one Creator whose name is Truth. Great is the ecstasy of that Supreme Wisdom

Ek	= One	Nam	= Identity
Ong	= Primal Vibration	Sïri	= Great
Kar	= Creation	Wahe	= Ecstasy
Sat	= Truth	Guru	= Wisdom

This is one of the first mantras Yogi Bhajan taught upon arrival to the U.S.A. **Ong** can also be defined as the *manifest creation*. This **Ashtang Mantra** balances the chakras & aura (7 chakras + 1 aura = 8 sounds).[9]
Asht = 8; Anga = Limb

WAH YANTI ~ *(7 minutes)*

Wah Yanti	Brahmadey
Kar Yanti	Treysha Guru
Jag Dūt Pati	Ït Wahe Guru
Adïk Ït Waha	

"Great Macroself, Creative Self, All that is creative through time, All that is the Great One, Three aspects of God: Brahma, Vishnu, Shiva; That is Wahe Guru"[10]

"This mantra is from the teachings of Patanjali. The practice of this mantra is the culmination of thousands of years of prayer."[11]

THE MUL MANTRA OF KUNDALINI YOGA ~ *(7 minutes)*

Ek Ong Kar	Seybang
Sat Nam	Gūr Prasad
Karta Purk	Jap
Nirbao	Aad Sach
Nir-ver	Jūgad Sach
Akal Mūrït	Heybi Sach
Ajūni	Nanïk Hosi Bi Sach

Ek Ong Kar	= One Creator, Creation
Sat Nam	= Truth is His/Her/God's Name
Karta Purk	= Doer of everything
Nirbao	= Fearless
Nir-ver	= Revengeless
Akal Mūrït	= Undying
Ajūni	= Unborn
Seybang	= Self Illumined
Gūr Prasad	= It is by Guru's Grace
Jap	= Recite through Repetition
Aad Sach	= True in the beginning
Jūgad Sach	= True through all the ages
Heybi Sach	= True even now
Nanïk Hosi Bi Sach	= Nanak says Truth shall ever be.

These were the first words spoken by Guru Nanak Dev Ji (1469-1593) upon his return from divine union. "Chanting this mantra helps you experience the depth and divinity of your soul. There are 108 elements in the universe and 108 letters in the mul mantra (in the original Gurmukhi script)."[12] **Mūl** means root, thus we call this the *Root Mantra* of Kundalini Yoga.

SAT SIRI SIRI AKAL ~ *Mantra for the Aquarian Age (7 minutes)*

Sat Sïri	= Great Truth,
Sïri Akal	= Great Undying
Sïri Akal	= Great Undying
Maha Akal	= Great Deathless
Maha Akal	= Great Deathless
Sat Nam	= Truth is the Name
Akal Mūrït	= Deathless Image of God
Wahe Guru	= This Wisdom is Bliss

Chanting this mantra connects you with the undying, eternal truth that is your true essence. "This mantra helps us to establish ourselves outside the change of time as deathless beings."[13]

RAK-E RAKANA HAR ~ *Final Verse from Rehiras Sahib of Guru Arjun Dev Ji (7 minutes)*

Rak-e Rakana-har Aap Ubarian
Gur Ki Peri Pai-e Kaj Savarian
Ho-a Aap Dai-al Manaho Na Visarian
Sad Jana Ke Sang Bavajal Tarian
Sakat Nïndak Dusht Kïn Ma-e Bïdarian
Tïs Sahïb Ki Teyk Nanïk Mane Ma-e
Jïs Sïmrat Sūk O-e Sagaley Dūk Ja-e

"The Protector Himself saves all. He causes us to fall at the feet of the Guru and fulfills the task. When He becomes merciful He does not forget the devotee. He provides means for the devotee to cross the world ocean by giving him the society of the True Saints. He destroys the non-believers and sinners in a moment. Nanak says, I take shelter of my master in my mind. By remembering Whom, bliss comes and all pains vanish." [14]

"This mantra adds energy to one's being and helps when you are physically weak. It does away with the obstacles to fulfilling one's destiny." [15]

WAHE GURU WAHE JIO ~ *(22 minutes)*

Wahe Guru
Wahe Guru
Wahe Guru
Wahe Jio

Wahe	= WOW, ecstasy
Guru	= Teacher, wisdom
Jio	= Beloved, soul
Gu	= Darkness, stickiness
Ru	= Remover of

Great Beyond Description is the experience of God's Wisdom...
Great Beyond Description is the experience of God The Beloved.

This is the mantra of ecstasy! "It expresses the indescribable experience of going from darkness to light." [16] **Waheguru** is also a term used in Punjabi that is synonomous with *God*.

GURU RAM DAS CHANT ~ *(5 minutes)*

Guru Guru Wahe Guru
Guru Ram Das Guru

This is a mantra of humility. [17] Chanting this mantra invokes the "spiritual light, guidance and protective grace" [18] of Guru Ram Das, the Fourth Sikh Guru. It opens the Fourth Chakra, the Heart Center, and allows you to feel and effortlessly radiate universal love.

This mantra was given to Yogi Bhajan through the subtle body of Guru Ram Das in India prior to his arrival to the West.

OTHER MANTRAS FROM KUNDALINI YOGA

AAD GUREY NAMEH
Please see Frequently Used Kundalini Yoga Mantras (pg. 2)

AAD SACH
Kundalini Shakti Mantra

Aad Sach	= True in the beginning
Jūgad Sach	= True through all the ages
Hey Bi Sach	= True even now
Nanïk Hosi Bi Sach	= Nanak says Truth shall ever be

"This mantra connects the speaker to the Infinite and the Infinite to the speaker."[19]

Aad Sach   Jūgad Sach   HeyBEY Sach   Nanïk Hosi BEY Sach

This is a slightly different permutation from the form above (HeyBEY [*hey bay*] replaces HeyBI [*hey bee*]). "When things do not move, this mantra adds the seeds of prosperity into your personality. All that is stuck shall move."[20]

AAP SAHAI HOA

Aap Sahai Hoa	= The Lord Him/Herself has become my protector
Sachey Da Sacha Doa	= The Truest of the True has taken care of me
Har Har Har	= God, God, God

"The Lord Him/Herself has become the protector; the Truest of the True has taken care of us, God, God God"[21]

"This mantra takes away negativity from the surrounding environments and from within. It is a gift that lets you penetrate into the unknown without fear. It gives protection and mental balance."[22]

ADEYS TISEY ADEYS
Please See Japji Sahib Section, 28 – 31st Pauri (pg. 50-Transliteration & pg. 60-Translation)

ADI MANTRA
For Individual Meditation[23]

Ong Namo Guru Deyv Namo Guru Deyv Namo Guru Deyv-a

I bow to the Divine Wisdom & Divine Teacher that is within My Self

"Use this mantra in its complete form anytime you have a lack of faith." "...when this mantra is chanted five times on one breath, the total spiritual knowledge of all teachers who have ever existed or who ever will exist on this earth, is beseated in that person."[24]

"If the limited individual ego in which we normally live is a small pond, then **Ong Namo** releases us into a vast and endless ocean. **Guru Deyv Namo** gives us the experience of the wisest seaman and all of his charts to guide us to the many ports we are to serve and experience."[25]

See also Ong Namo Guru Deyv Namo (pg. 1)

ADI SHAKTI
Kundalini Bhakti Mantra

Adi Shakti, Namo Namo	= I bow to the Primal Power (Feminine)
Sarab Shakti, Namo Namo	= I bow to the All-Encompassing Energy
Prītam Bagvati, Namo Namo	= I bow to that through which God creates
Kūndalini Mata Shakti, Namo Namo	= I bow to the creative power of Kundalini

"This devotional mantra invokes the primary creative Power which is manifest as the feminine. It helps one to become free of insecurities."[26]

'I call upon the ***Power of Divine Mother***.' *Mata Shakti* is the Sacred Feminine. **Namo** represents the act of bowing and the embodiment of humility.

AJAI ALAI
Verses 189-196 from Jap Sahib of Guru Gobind Singh (pg. 87)

Ajai Alai Abhai Abai	= Invincible, Indestructible, Fearless, Immortal
Abū Ajū Anas Akas	= Unborn, Forever, Indestructible, All-pervading
Aganj Abanj Alak Abak	= Invincible, Indivisible, Invisible, Free of wants
Akal Deyal Aleyk Abeyk	= Immortal, Kind, Unimaginable, Formless
Anam, Akam	= Unnameable, Desireless,
Agaha, Adaha	= Unfathomable, Undamageable
Anatey, Parmatey	= Without a Master, Destroyer of All
Ajoni, Amoni	= Beyond Birth & Death, Beyond Silence
Na Ragey, Na Rangey	= More than Love itself, Beyond all Colors
Na Rūpey Na Reykey	= Formless, Beyond Chakras
Akaramang, Agaramang	= Beyond Karma, Beyond Doubt
Aganjey, Aleykey	= Beyond Battlers, Unimaginable

Ajai Alai is a mantra which rouses the soul and the self. "It brings great sensitivity to the Being and gives the ability to be able to compute what people are actually saying automatically. Once you recite this mantra correctly, it will give you the power that whatever you say must happen. When you chant this mantra you have the power to surpass anything."[27]

Alternative pronunciation for Line 1: **Ajey Aley Abhey Abey**

AKAL
The Great Undying

This mantra is a powerful life-giving chant that serves to remove fear and relax the mind. It may be chanted at length to serve the transition of the soul of a friend or loved one. This is done by extending the sounds of the word for the duration of a complete breath. Inhale deeply and chant 'Ah' then a long drawn out 'Kaaal' for the length of the breath, enunciating the 'L' sound at the end. This mantra serves in sending the soul back *home*. It is a great gift to a soul that has left the body.

"Akal means *timelessness* and timelessness means *deathlessness*."[28]

AKAN JOR
Please see Japji Sahib, 33rd Pauri (pg. 51-Transliteration & pg. 61-Translation)

ALAK BABA SÏRI CHAND DÏ-RAK

This mantra calls upon Baba Sïri Chand, the first son of Guru Nanak Dev Ji and master of the ascetic Udasi sect of Yogis from India. This mantra deflects the negativity of a psychic attack.

IT IS ONLY TO BE CHANTED ONCE PER DAY.[29]

Alak means *invisible* or *unseen*.

ANAND
Verse 1 from Anand Sahib of Guru Amar Das (pg. 102)

> **Anand Bai-a Meyri Ma-i Satïguru Mey Pai-a**
> **Satïgur Ta Pa-ia Sahej Seyti Man Vaji-a Vadha-ia**
> **Rag Ratan Parvar Pari-a Shabd Gavana-ia**
> **Shabado Ta Gavaho Hari Keyra Manjïni Vasa-ia**
> **Kahey Nanïk Anand Ho-a Satïguru Mey Pa-ia**

"I am in ecstasy, O my mother, for I have found my True Guru. I have found the True Guru, with intuitive ease & my mind vibrates with the music of bliss. The jeweled melodies & their celestial harmonies have come to sing the Word of the Shabd. The

Lord dwells within the minds of those who sing the Shabd. Says Nanak, I am in ecstasy, for I have found my True Guru."[30]

It is widely believed among Sikhs that who ever recites the forty *pauris*, or stanzas, of *Anand* will have endless bliss. This *Bani*, or prayer, can be read in it's entirety on pg. 103.

ANAND SAHIB
Please see Anand Sahib Section (pg. 102)

ANG SANG WAHE GURU
From Guru Amar Das, 3rd Master of the Sikhs

> **Ang Sang Wahe Guru**

Each and every cell of my being is vibrating with the ecstasy of the Divine

Ang	= Limb or part of a body, or the body itself – the part
Sang	= Union, association – the whole
Wahe	= Ecstasy, WOW
Guru	= That which takes us from darkness to light

"This mantra eliminates haunting thoughts."[31]

ANT-NA SIFTI
Please see Japji Sahib Section, 24th Pauri (pg. 48-Transliteration & pg. 58 Translation)

ARDAS BAHI

> Ardas Ba-hi Amar Das Guru
> Amar Das Guru Ardas Ba-hi
> Ram Das Guru Ram Das Guru
> Ram Das Guru Sachi Sahïb

The prayer has been given to Guru Amar Das (3rd Sikh Master)
The prayer is manifested by Guru Ram Das (4th Sikh Master)
The miracle is complete

"This is a simple permutation and combination of words that manifests beyond the realm of creativity and activity. Chant this mantra to help release a difficult situation. Ardas Ba-hi is a mantra of prayer. If you sing it, automatically, without having to say what you want, the need of life is adjusted."[32]

AVAL ALLAH
Poem by By Kabir from Siri Guru Granth Sahib

Aval Ala Nur Upai-a Kūdarat Ke Sab Bandey
Ek Nur Te Sab Jag Upajeya Kūn Bal-e Ko Mandey
Loga Baram Na Būlahu Ba-i
Khalek Khalek Khalek Mehi Khalik Por Reho Sarab Ta-i
Mati Ek Anek Bant Kar Saji Sajanaharey
Na Kach Poch Mati Ke Bandey Na Kach Poch Kūnbarey
Sab Mehi Sacha Eko So-i Tis Ka Kia Sab Kech Ho-i
Hūkam Pachaney So Eko Janey Banda Kahi-ey So-i
Alo Alak Na Jai-i Lakia Gur Gura Dina Mita
Kahe Kabir Meri Sanka Nasi Sarab Niranjan Dita

"First, Allah created the Light; then, by His Creative Power, He made all mortal beings. From the One Light, the entire universe welled up. So, who is good and who is bad? O people, O Siblings of Destiny, do not wander deluded by doubt. The Creation is in the Creator, and the Creator is in the Creation, totally pervading and permeating all places. The clay is the same, but the Fashioner has fashioned it in various ways. There is nothing wrong with the pot of clay - there is nothing wrong with the Potter. The One True Lord abides in all; by His making, everything is made. Whoever realizes the *Hukam* of His Command, knows the One Lord. He alone is said to be the Lord's slave. The Lord Allah is Unseen; He cannot be seen. The Guru has blessed me with this sweet molasses. Says Kabir, my anxiety and fear have been taken away; I see the Immaculate Lord pervading everywhere."[33]

AAAA-OOOO-UMMM
Nad Meditation Mantra: Nad Namodam Rasa[34]

Aaaa – Oooo – Ummm

Aaaa	= Represents 'Come'
Oooo	= Represents 'Thou'
Ummm	= Represents 'We'

"Come, Thou, into the form of Life"

This mantra can be used to facilitate communication prior to a meeting. In the Kundalini Yoga tradition, this mantra is not chanted as OM, but rather, as three distinct, but blended, sounds. Yogi Bhajan called this a *Trikuti Mantra*, in that it blends all 3 *Gunas* (the 3 qualities of *Maya*, or illusion of reality).

The 3 Gunas bind the soul to the material world; they are:

Satva – Purity which binds the soul with happiness and knowledge
Rajas – Passion or Desire which bind the soul through attachment
Tamas – Darkness which binds the soul with power, recklessness and selfishness.

BA-OTA KARAM
Japji Sahib, 25th Pauri (pg. 49-Transliteration & pg. 58-Translation)

BOLO RAM

Bolo = Sing!
Ram = Ram is the 7th incarnation of Vishnu

Everybody sing aloud, Ram!

"Ram literally means one who is divinely blissful and who gives joy to others; one in whom the sages rejoice"[35]

BOLE SONIHAL – DEYH SHIVA
From Dasam Granth Sahib of Guru Gobind Singh

Boley So Nihal	He who speaks (this) will be blessed
Sat Sïri Akal!	The Truth is Great and Undying!
Dey Shiva Bar Mo-eh I-hey	Grant me, O God, this blessing
Shab Karaman Tey Kabahū Na Taron	May I never refrain from righteous acts
Na Daro Ar So Jab Jai Laro	May I fearlessly fight all foes in battle
Nisachey Kar Apani Jit Karo	With the courage of Faith, achieve Victory
Ar Sïkh Hao Apaney Hi Man Kao	Ingrain my mind with Your Teachings
Ih Lalach Hau Gun Tau Ucharo	May my ambition be to sing Your Praises
Jab Aav Ki Aud Nidan Baney	And, when this mortal life comes to its end
At Hi Ran Mey Tab Jūj Maro	May I die fighting, with limiltess courage
Jau Tau Preym Key-lan Ka Cha-o	If you desire to play the game of love, then
Sir Dar Tali Gali Meyri Aa-o	Place your head in palm, come onto my path
Ït Marag Peyr Dari-jey	On this road, place your feet
Sir Di-jey Kan Na Ki-jey	Offer your head, pay no mind to opinions
Sūra So Pehichani-ey	He alone is known as a warrior hero
Jo Larey Din Key Heyt	Who fights for the sake of religion
Purja purja Kat Marey	Limb by limb he may be cut apart and killed
Kabahū Na Chadey Keyt	But he will never desert the battlefield
Marta Marta Jag Mū-a	People die in the world everyday
Mar Bi Na Jani Ko-i	But they do not know how to truly die
Eysey Marney Jo Marey	Whoever dies, let him die such a death
Bahur Na Marna Ho-i	That he shall not have to die again
Boley So Nihal	He who speaks will be blessed
Sat Sïri Akal!	The Truth is Great and Undying![36]

This comes from the writings of Guru Gobind Singh, the 10th and last of the Sikh Masters. This pays honor to those who gave their lives in the Name of Truth. It is a ballad for the defender of peace and freedom as well as the spiritual warrior.

BOUNTIFUL, BLISSFUL, BEAUTIFUL

> I am Bountiful, Blissful and Beautiful
> Bountiful, Blissful and Beautiful I am

or

Bountiful am I, Blissful am I, Beautiful am I

"This is a mantra for the affirmation and strengthening of self-esteem and self-confidence." The following version of the mantra is called *Mantra of Bliss: Affirmation of the Divine Self*[37].

The Mantra of Bliss contains the first part of Anand Sahib (translation pg. 8). It also contains the mantra *Ek Ong Kar Sat Gur Prasad* (Siri Mantra) "which elevates the self beyond duality and establishes the flow of spirit"[38] (translation pg. 16).

> I am Bountiful, Blissful and Beautiful
> Bountiful, Blissful and Beautiful I am
> Ek Ong Kar Sat Gur Prasad
> Anand Bai-a Meyri Ma-i Satiguru Mey Pai-a
> Satigur Ta Pa-ia Sahej Seyti Man Vaji-a Vadha-ia
> Rag Ratan Parvar Pari-a Shabd Gavana-ia
> Shabado Ta Gavaho Hari Keyra Manjini Vasa-ia
> Kahey Nanik Anand Ho-a Satiguru Mey Pa-ia

BY THY GRACE
Words by Yogi Bhajan & Snatam Kaur[39]

> It's by Thy Grace that I sing Your Holy Name
> It's by Thy Grace that I feel Your Holy Name
> One day the day shall come when all the Glory shall be Thine
> People will say it is yours and I shall deny, 'not mine'
> Peace to all, Life to all, Love to all

CHAKRA CHIHN
Verse 1 from Jap Sahib of Guru Gobind Singh (pg. 71)

> Chakra Chihn Ar Baran Jat Ar Pat Nehin Je
> Rūp Rang Ar Reyk Beyk Ku-ke-na Sakat Ke
> Achal Mūrat Anabo Prakash Amitoj Kahe-jey
> Kot Indr Indran Sahu Sahan Gane-jey
> Tri-bavan Mahip Sur Nar Asur Net Net Ban Tren Kahet
> Tav Sarab Nam Kate Kavan Karam Nam Baranat Sumat

"God is such a being who is without any caste, class or mark
God's form, outline and color are indescribable

Unchanging, self-illuminated, with immense power
King of millions of Indras (King of gods), King of kings, God of the three worlds
Even the earth's green plants announce that none is equal to God
None can describe all of the names of God
The wise sing the names according to her/his attributes, excellences & works"[40]

CHARN SAT SAT
Astpadi-17, Verse 1 from Sukhmani Sahib of Guru Arjun Dev Ji

Charn Sat Sat Parsan-har	Ape Gūn Ape Gūn Kari
Pūja Sat Sat Seva-dar	Shabd Sat Sat Prab Bakta
Darshan Sat Sat Pekan-har	Surat Sat Sat Jas Sūnta
Nam Sat Sat Diavan-har	Būjan-har Kau Sat Sab Ho-e
Aap Sat Sat Sab Dari	Nanïk Sat Sat Prab So-e

"God's feet are true and those touching them, also true
His worship is true and his worshippers, also true
His sight is true and his beholders, also true
His name is true and those who meditate on it, also true
He Himself is true and all that He sustains are true
He Himself is virtuous and Himself bestower of virtues
His Word is true and the reciter of the word, also true
Meditation on God's Name is true and those who hear the praises of God, also true
Those who realize Him, for them all is truth
O, Nanak, true, true is God"[41]

CHATR CHAKR VARTI
Verse 199 (Last Four Lines) from Jap Sahib of Guru Gobind Singh (pg. 88)

Chatr Chakr Varti	Dū-kalang Pranasi
Chatr Chakr Bū-gatey	Dey-alang Sarūpey
Sū-yambav Sūbang	Sada-ang Sangey
Sarab Da Sarab Jū-gatey	Abang-ang Bï-būtey

"God is present on all sides and by His Order controls all the world. God's Light is automatic; He is beautiful and is ever present in all living beings. God destroys the pains of births and deaths, and is the embodiment of mercy. God is present with all and His grandeur will never vanish."[42]

"These are the final lines of *Jap Sahib*. This mantra removes fear, anxiety, depression, & phobias as it brings victory. It instills courage & fearlessness into the fiber of the person. It gives *sahibi* (control over one's domain), self-command & self-grace. Recite it when your position is endangered; when your authoritative personality is weak."[43]

CHARDI KALA
Prayer from Ardas of Guru Gobind Singh and Successors

Nanïk Nam Chardi Kala Tere Bane Sarbat Da Pala

O God, In the Name of Nanak, may your name forever be exalted to bring prosperity to all beings

Nanïk Nam = In the Name of Nanak   **Tere Bane** = The will or pleasure of God
Chardi Kala = The Ever-rising Spirit   **Sarbat Da Pala** = Blessings for All

"**Chardi Kala** signifies a perennially blossoming, unwilting spirit; a perpetual state of certitude resting on the unwavering belief in Divine justice. The **Kala,** of Sanskrit origin, gives a powerful notation which is 'Energy'. **Chardi**, in Punjabi, means *rising* or *ascending. Chardi Kala* simply means a Rising Spirit in an intensely energized, ever-ascending state. It is characterized by faith, confidence, discipline and readiness to perform the assigned tasks even in the face of the most daunting challenge."[44]

"If you want to have an equal literary meaning to this, this only means 'Rising Spirit'. In other words, if you have a Christian background, it is called 'resurrection'."[45]

DHAN DHAN RAM DAS GURU
Shabd by Satte and Balvand from Siri Guru Granth Sahib

Dhan Dhan Ram Das Guru Jïn Sïria Tïney Savari-a
Pūri Ho-i Karamat Aap Sirjan-harey Dari-a
Sïki Atey Sangati Parbrahm Kar Namasakari-a
Atal Ataho Atol Tu Teyra Ant Na Paravari-a
Jïni Tu Seyvi-a Ba-o Kar Sey Tūd Par Utari-a
Lab Lob Kam Krod Moho Mar Kadey Tūd Saparvari-a
Dhan So Teyra Tan Hey Sach Teyra Peyskari-a
Nanïk Tu Leyna Tu Hey Guru Amar Tu Vichari-a
Gur Dïta Ta Man Sadhari-a

"Praise unto Ram Das the Guru, the one who created you, established you. You are such a miracle! The creator has installed you on a throne. Your Sikhs (Students), & all conscious people bow to you because you manifest God. You are unchanging, unfathomable, and immeasurable. Your limit cannot be perceived. Those who serve you with love are carried across the sea of existence. The 5 obstacles (greed, attachment, lust, anger, ego) cannot exist where you are. The realm that you rule is the true place. This is your glory. You are Nanak, Angad, and Amar Das the Guru. Oh, when I recognized you, my soul was comforted!"[46]

"This shabd reaches the realm of miracles. The impossible becomes possible. It is the realm of the heart, the Neutral Mind, where all things become pure."[47]

DHARTI HAE
2008 3HO Global Meditation: Earth Tatva - Isht Shodhana Kriya Mantra[48]

Dharti (or Pritvi) Hae	= Earth Is
Akash Hae	= Heaven Is
Guru Ram Das Hae	= The Neutral Mind (Aspect of Guru Ram Das) Is

"**Isht** means to have the solidified God realization. **Shodhana** is to straighten out. This mantra is to be chanted during the falling of the sun, not in the morning, in order to attain the Siddhi, or yogic power of knowing, the vision of time and space."[49]

It can be chanted with either the sound '*Pritvi*' or '*Darti*' as Earth though '*Darti*' is taught for the kriya.

DUK PAR HAR
Please see Japji Sahib Section, 5th Pauri (pg. 45-Transliteration & pg. 54-Translation)

EK ONG KAR-AH
Laya Yoga Mantra of Kundalini Yoga[50] *(Adi Shakti Mantra)*

There is one Creator whose name is Truth
Great is the ecstasy of that Supreme Wisdom

Ek Ong Kar-AH
Sat-a Nam-AH
Sïri Wa-AH
-he Guru

Ek	= One	**Nam**	= Identity
Ong	= Primal Vibration	**Sïri**	= Great
Kar	= Creation	**Wahe**	= Ecstasy
Sat	= Truth	**Guru**	= Wisdom

"This mantra brings the soul and destiny present. It suspends you above conflicts attracted by success and the activity of the Positive mind."[51]

The articulation of the mantra is done in a cycle of 3 ½. The 'AH' sound is created by firmly lifting the diaphragm rather than from the voice. There is a brief pause following each 'AH' but no pause between '*he Guru*' and '*Ek Ong Kar*' as the mantra is repeated.

According to Hatha Yoga Pradipika, "**Laya** refers to the dissolution of the mind and **Laya Yoga** is the attainment of Supreme Consciousness through devotion."[52]

EK ONG KAR SAT GUR PRASAD
Siri Mantra

> Ek Ong Kar Sat Gur Prasad
> Sat Gur Prasad Ek Ong Kar

Ek	= One
Ong	= Infinite creative energy in manifestation
Kar	= The Creation
Sat	= Truth
Gur	= Teacher, which takes us from dark to light
Prasad	= Gift

"God and We are One. I know this by the Grace of the True Guru.
I know this by the Grace of the True Guru. That God and We are One."[53]

"This mantra is a *gutka shabd* - one that reverses the mind. It needs to be chanted with reverence, in a place of reverence. After chanting this mantra, anything you say will be amplified with great force. So have a positive projection and do not say anything negative for a while."[54] **Gur Prasad** means *Gift of the Guru.*

EK ONG KAR SAT NAM SIRI WAHE GURU
Sex Energy Transformation Kriya Mantra[55]

There is one Creator whose name is Truth. Great is the ecstasy of that Supreme Wisdom.

Ek	= One	Nam	= Identity
Ong	= Primal Vibration	Sïri	= Great
Kar	= Creation	Wahe	= Ecstasy
Sat	= Truth	Guru	= Wisdom

This mantra (when done according to the instructions of Sex Energy Transformation Kriya) "uses the Kundalini energy to project the mind into the infinity of the cosmos and beyond the normal earthly consciousness."[56]

ETERNO SOL
Long Time Sun (Spanish)

Que El Eterno Sol Te Ilumine	= May the eternal sun illuminate you
Que El Amor Te Rodee	= May Love surround you
Y La Luz Pura Interior	= And the pure light within
Guie Tu Camino	= Guide your way; path, journey

"May the Long Time Sun shine upon you, all Love surround you, And the Pure Light within you, Guide your way on."[57]

GANAPATI MANTRA
Panj Shabd with Siri Gaitri Mantra

Sa Ta Na Ma Ra Ma Da Sa Sa Sey So Hang

Sa	= Infinity, cosmos, beginning		**Da**	= Earth
Ta	= Life, existence		**Sa**	= Impersonal Infinity
Na	= Death, change, transformation		**Sa**	= Impersonal Infinity
Ma	= Rebirth		**Sey**	= Thou
Ra	= Sun		**So**	= Personal sense of identity
Ma	= Moon		**Hang**	= The Infinite, vibrating, real
Sa+Sey	= Totality of Infinity		**So+Hang**	= I Am Thou

This is a mantra for "Making the Impossible Possible"[58]. Its full effects are achieved when done in the form of Ganpati Kriya Meditation as taught by Yogi Bhajan.[59]

GOBINDA HARI

Gobïnda Gobïnda Hari Hari

Gobïnda = The sustainer, support for/of all
Hari = The beautiful, potent, healing God

The common transliteration from *Sankrit* is spelled Govinda, with a V; Gobinda, with a B from *Punjabi*.

GOBINDEY MUKANDEY
Guru Gaitri Mantra (also know as Sarab Shakti Mantra)

Gobïndey	= Sustaining		**Hariang**	= Destroying
Mūkandey	= Liberating		**Kariang**	= Creating
Udarey	= Enlightening		**Nirnamey**	= Nameless
Aparey	= Infinite		**Akamey**	= Desireless

"This mantra can eliminate karmic blocks or errors of the past. It has the power to purify one's magnetic field, making it easier to relax and meditate. It is a protective mantra, an ashtang mantra (having 8 parts). Besides cleansing the subconscious mind, it balances the hemispheres of the brain, bringing compassion and patience to the one who meditates on it."[60]

GOD AND ME

God and Me, Me and God Are One[61]

This English affirmation from Yogi Bhajan reminds us that we need look nowhere but within to find the living God.

GURU DEYV MATA
Shabd by Guru Arjun Dev Ji from Siri Guru Granth Sahib

Guru Deyv Mata
The Divine Teacher is our mother
Guru Deyv Pïta
The Divine Teacher is our father
Guru Deyv Swami Parmeysarey
...our Master; The Transcendent Lord
Guru Deyv Saka Agian Banjan
...my companion; the destroyer of ignorance
Guru Deyv Bandïp Sahodara
...my relative and brother
Guru Deyv Data Har Nam Upadeysey
 ...the giver; teacher of the Lord's Name
Guru Deyv Mantr Nirodara
...the infallible mantra
Guru Deyv Sant Sat Būd Mūrat
...the image of peace, truth and wisdom
Guru Deyv Paras Paras Para
 ...magic; touching it one is transformed
Guru Deyv Tirat Amrït Sarovar
...sacred shrine of pilgrimage; pool of divine nectar
Guru Gian Majan Aparampara
Bathing in wisdom, one experiences the Infinite
Guru Deyv Karta Sab Pap Harta
...the Creator and the Destroyer of all sins
Guru Deyv Patït Pavït Kara
...purifier of the impure
Guru Deyv Aad Jugad Jug Jug
...existed in the beginning & throughout the ages
Guru Deyv Mantr Har Jap Udara
...the enlightening mantra of the Lords' Name
Guru Deyv Sangat Prab Meyla Kar Kirpa
...the merciful, permitting me into this society
Ham Mūr Papi Jït Lag Tara
I am foolish, but holding onto this, I will be carried
Guru Deyv Sat Gur Parabram Parameysarey
...the True Guru, the Supreme Transcendent Lord
Guru Deyv Nanïk Har Namaskara
Nanak bows in humble reverence to the Lord[62]

GURU RAM DAS
2011 3HO Global Meditation - Air Tatva Meditation Mantra[63]
Please see Aquarian Sadhana Mantras Section (pg. 5)

GURU RAM DAS RAKO SARANA-I
From Kirat, the Poet

> ### Guru Ram Das Rako Sarana-i
>
> "Guru Ram Das, protect me and surround me with your Sanctuary"[64]
>
> **Rako** = To keep, protect   **Sarana-i** = Salvation
>
> Guru Ram Das was the 4th Sikh Master and the etheric Guru of Yogi Bhajan. He is considered to be like a Patron Saint of Kundalini Yoga as Taught by Yogi Bhajan® as well as a bestower of miracles.

GURU SAT GURU
From Siri Guru Granth Sahib

> ### Guru Sat Guru Kajo Sïk Akai-ey
> ### So Bal Key ūta Har Nam Di-avey
>
> "One who considers her/his self to be a disciple of the True Guru, should rise before the coming of the light and contemplate the Name."[65]
>
> This mantra summarizes one of Yogi Bhajans most basic teachings: wake up before the sun rises for your Sadhana (daily practice).

HAM DAM HAR HAR

> **Ham Dam Har Har   Har Har Ham Dam**
>
> We are the Universe, God, God. God, God, the Universe are We.
>
> **Ham**   = Creative essence of the person
> **Dam**   = Pranic essence of the person
> **Har**   = Creative essence of God
>
> "This mantra opens the Heart Chakra, the center of compassion."[66]

HA-MI HAM BRAHM HAM
We are We, We are God

> ### Ha-mi Ham Brahm Ham
>
> **Ha-mi Ham**   = I am Thine
> **Brahm**   = The Supreme Consciousness
> **Ham**   = Creative essence of the person
>
> "This mantra literally means that we are the spirit of God. It is total spirit. Total spirit represents God. It fixes the identity into its true reality."[67]

HA-MI HAM TU-MI TUM
2013 3HO Global Meditation: First Sutra[68]

Ha-mi Ham	= I am Thine
Tū-mi Tūm	= In mine myself
Wahe Guru	= Ecstasy beyond words

I am Thine, in mine, Myself, Wahe Guru (in the experience of Divine Ecstasy)

HAR

Har	= Creative Infinite aspect of God

Har is a sound of the heart. It has the potential to clear blocks that may prevent prosperity and success. This sound appears in countless kriyas and meditations within the technology of Kundalini Yoga as Taught by Yogi Bhajan®. The mantra is chanted by strongly pulling in and up on the navel point. The 'r' is produced by flicking the tip of the tongue to the roof of the mouth, just behind the front teeth.

HAR GOBIND MAHAN HAE

Har Gobïnd Har Gobïnd Har Gobïnd Mahan Hae
Sarab Shakti Sarab Shakti Sarab Shakti Mahan Hae

Great is God, The One which sustains us; Great is this all-encompassing Divine Feminine

Har	= Creative Infinite aspect of God
Gobïnda	= The sustainer, support for/of all
Mahan	= Great
Sarab	= All Encompassing
Shakti	= Divine Feminine Energy
Hae	= Is

HAR HAR HAR AMRITSAR

Har	= Creative, Infinite aspect of God
Amritsar	= Sacred City, where the Sikh Golden Temple is

Chanting this mantra is meant to invoke the essence of the healing and holy waters that surround the Golden Temple.[69]

Amrit literally means nectar.

HAR HAR HAR HAR GOBINDEY
Guru Gaitri Mantra with 4 Hars

Har Har Har Har Gobïndey	= God, Sustaining
Har Har Har Har Mūkandey	= God, Liberating
Har Har Har Har Udarey	= God, Enlightening
Har Har Har Har Aparey	= God, Infinite
Har Har Har Har Hariang	= God, Destroying
Har Har Har Har Kariang	= God, Creating
Har Har Har Har Nirnamey	= God, Nameless
Har Har Har Har Akamey	= God, Desireless

"This is a mantra that fixes the mind to prosperity and power. It invokes guidance and sustenance."[70]

Har is the name of God; the Creative, Infinite aspect. It is a sound of the heart. It has the potential to clear blocks that may prevent prosperity and success.

HAR HAR HAR HAR HARINAM

Har	= Creative Infinite aspect of God
Harinam	= The manifestation of infinite creativity in action

HAR HAR MUKANDEY

Har	= Creative, Infinite aspect of God
Mūkandey	= Liberating aspect of Self

"This mantra turns challenges into opportunities; removes fear."[71]

HAR HAR RAM DAS GURU HAE

Har	= Creative Infinite aspect of God
Guru Ram Das	= 4th Master of the Sikhs
Hae	= Is

Through the subtle body of Baba Siri Chand this mantra was given to Sunder Singh as his personal mantra in a very challenging time of his life (early 70's). He received the blessing of Yogi Bhajan to teach it, as it was a *'gift from Guru Ram Das'*. 30 years later, he requested that Snatam Kaur record it.[72] By account, this mantra has the potential to turn one's life around. In the darkest night, the grace of Guru Ram Das manifests with this mantra. Guru Ram Das is like a Patron Saint of Kundalini Yoga.

Ram is the 7th incarnation of Vishnu though the word is commonly used as a sound for God. **Das** literally means *'One who Serves'*. Together, **Ram Das** is *'The One Who Serves God'*.

HAR HAR WAHE GURU

Har, Har	= Creative Infinite aspect of God
Wahe	= WOW, ecstasy
Guru	= Remover of Darkness; which takes us from darkness to light

"Chanting this mantra creates balance between the earth and ether and eliminates subconscious blocks from the past, particularly father/mother phobias."[73]

HAR HAREY HARI WAHE GURU

Har	= Creative Infinite aspect of God (*Masc.*)
Harey	= Flowing aspect of God (*Neutral*)
Hari	= Creation in Action (*Fem.*)
Wahe	= WOW, ecstasy
Guru	= Remover of Darkness; which takes us from darkness to light

"This is both a Shakti and Bhakti mantra. It expresses the three aspects of the sound *Har*: seed, flow & completion unto the infinite. It can bring you through any block in life."[74]

HAR HARI
Guru Nanak's Treasure Meditation Mantra[75]

Har Har Har Har Hari Hari

Har = Creative Infinite aspect of God   **Hari** = Creation in Action

When done in the meditation form, each *Har* is one beat and each *Hari* is two beats, for a total of 8.

"This (mantra) meditation builds a deep sense of self-reliance. It allows you to separate your identity from your success. It gives you potency, productivity, and caliber. It makes you experience and believe in yourself so that success comes to serve you, rather than you running after it."[76]

HAR JI
Mantra for Breaking Through the Mask[77]

Har Ji Har Har   Har Har Har Ji

Oh, my Beloved (soul), God, God, God, God is my Beloved (soul)

Har = God (Creative Infinite Aspect)   **Ji** = Beloved, soul

"These sounds manifest from the Infinite subtlety of God into immediate experience. It opens your soul to be real and your mind to link effectively to your real identity. Along with the mudra, its subtle and electromagnetic form adjusts the projection of the heart center and lets your words go deeply into your mind to guide your new behaviors."[78]

HAR KA NAM
From Basant Ki Var of Guru Arjun Dev Ji

> Har Ka Nam Dia-ey Key Hohu Hari-a Ba-I
> Karam Likantey Pai-ey-ïh Rūt Suha-I

"Contemplate God's Name in accordance with the writ of destiny & blossom forth in green abundance. By your high destiny you have been blessed with this wondrous spring of the soul."[79]

This mantra of gratitude is for calling in or blessing another with abundance and prosperity.

HAR SINGH NAR SINGH

> Har Sïng Nar Sïng Nil Narayan Guru Sïk Guru Sïng Har Har Gyan
> Wahe Guru Wahe Guru Gar Gar Di-an Sakat Nïndak Dusht Matayan

"God the Protector takes care of the universe. Those who live in God-consciousness and power, chant *Har Har*. Meditate on *Wahe Guru* and live in ecstasy. For those who vibrate God's name and relate to God, all karmas are cleared."[80]

This mantra works to strengthen the masculine energy and it has the power to dispel evil. **Singh** is commonly translated as *lion*.

HAR WAHE GURU SAT NAM HAR HARI
Mantra Meditation to Experience Your Own Soul Blessing You with Prosperity[81]

> Har Har Har Har Wahe Guru Sat Nam Har Hari

Har	= Creative Infinite aspect of God
Wahe	= WOW, ecstasy
Guru	= That which takes us from darkness to light
Sat	= Truth
Nam	= Identity
Har	= Creative Infinite aspect of God
Hari	= Creation in Action

This particular sequence and permutation can elevate your energy so that you can more easily experience your own soul blessing you with prosperity. In the meditation form, visualizations are taking place from the 3rd Chakra to the 7th Chakra.

HARI NAM SAT NAM
God's name is the name of Truth

Hari Nam Sat Nam Hari Nam Hari, Hari Nam Sat Nam Sat Nam Hari

Hari Nam	= God's Name
Sat Nam	= Truth's Name
Hari	= Creation in Action
Sat	= Truth
Nam	= Identity, Name

This mantra is both heart-opening and for prosperity.

I AM I AM
Mantra Meditation Into Being: "I Am, I Am"[82]

"The first *I AM* is the personal, finite sense of self. The second *I AM* is the impersonal and Infinite Self. If you only say the first *I AM* the mind will automatically try to answer, '*I am what?* This sends the mind on a search through all the categories and roles that hold the finite identities. If you immediately say the second part of the mantra, *I AM* the thought becomes *I AM What I AM.*"

To *BE WHAT YOU BE* is the essence of truth and will lead you to the nature of Reality.

I AM HAPPY, I AM GOOD
"I Am Happy" Mantra Meditation for Children[83]

I am Happy, I am Good
I am Happy, I am Good
Sat Nam Sat Nam Sat Nam Ji
Wahe Guru Wahe Guru Wahe Guru Ji

Sat	= Truth
Nam	= Identity, Name
Ji	= Beloved, soul
Wahe	= WOW, ecstasy
Guru	= Teacher, wisdom

This meditation was given by Yogi Bhajan for children to experience the power of words, mantras and affirmations, particularly in times of crisis or when parents are fighting.

I AM THE LIGHT OF MY SOUL

I Am The Light Of My Soul
I Am Beautiful I Am Bountiful
I Am Bliss I Am I Am

JAP MAN SAT NAM
Shabd by Guru Amar Das from Siri Guru Granth Sahib

Jap Man Sat Nam Sada Sat Nam

Oh my Mind, Repeat the vibration of *Sat Nam*, The True Name

Jap	= Recite through repetition
Man	= Mind
Sat Nam	= Truth is Thy Name
Sada	= Constant, eternal
Sat Nam	= Truth is Thy Name

"This mantra opens up the flow of prosperity by attuning the mind to the power *Har*, the Creative Infinity, the Joy of merger with the Infinity."[84]

JAP SAHIB
Please see Jap Sahib Section (pg. 71)

JAPJI SAHIB
Please see Japji Sahib Section (pg. 43)

JEI TE GANG
From Dasam Granth Sahib of Guru Gobind Singh

Jei Jei Jag Karan Srist ūbaran Mam Prïtïparan Jei Tegang, Jei Jei Tegang
Kag Kand Bihandan Kal Dal Kandan At Ran Mandan Bar Bandan
Būj Dand Akandan Teyj Parchandan Jot Amandan Ban Praban
Sūk Santa Karnang Durmat Darnang Kilbïk Harnang As Sarnang

"The sword breaks through and cuts down the demons of the mind and body. This beautiful and powerful weapon adorns the battlefield of life. It is as an extension of the arm; unbreakable, terribly fast; its awesome splendor overshadows even the sun. It protects the peace and happiness of the saints and destroys any powerful negative energy. It has erased the negativity and guilt that I carry. I seek its refuge. Praise, praise be to the great Doer of the world, savior of the creation, my great protector; praise be to the sword!"[85]

This mantra "cuts around karma"[86] and "can cut through any negativity"[87]. It is serves to give one courage and self-esteem.

JIN PREMA KIO
Verse 9 from Tav Prasad Svaye of Guru Gobind Singh (pg. 99)

Jïn Prema Kio Tïn Hi Prab Pay-o
Sach Ke-o Sūn Leyo Sab-ey
Kaha Beyo Jo Do Lochan Mūnd Key
Bet Rai-o Bak Dian Lagay-o
Nat Firio Li-ey Sat Samundran
Lok Geyo Perlok Gavey-o
Bas Ki-o Bïkian So Bet-key
Asey He Asey So Beys Bïtai-o
Sach Ke-o Sūn Leyo Sab-ey
Jïn Prema Kio Tïn Hi Prab Pay-o

Only the one who is absorbed in True Love (*Prema*) shall attain the Lord. I speak the Truth. Listen and understand completely. Amongst fear and the noise of the mind's chatter, remain sitting with both eyes closed in meditation. Though you bathe at Holy places and wander the seven seas, this world is lost and the next world is lost when you wander away from the seat of your own heart. The yogi sits among distraction, difficulties and illusion, and in this way of sitting still, the strength of the spirit emerges. I speak the Truth. Listen and understand completely. Only the one who is absorbed in True Love shall attain the Lord. [88]

KAL AKAL

Kal Akal Sïri Akal, Maha Akal Akal Mūrït

Kal	= Death
Akal	= Undying, Deathless
Sïri	= Powerful
Akal	= Undying, Deathless
Maha	= Great
Akal	= Undying, Deathless
Mūrït	= Image of God
Kal Akal	= Death/Deathless
Siri Akal	= Great Undying
Maha Akal	= Great Deathless
Akal Mūrït	= Deathless Image of God

This mantra is chanted for the removal of the shadow of death. It also works to seal animosity, rendering it ineffective.

KAURI KRIYA MANTRA[89]
Sargam, Panj Shabd & Siri Gaitri Mantra

> Sa Rey Ga Ma Pa Da Ni
> Sa Ta Na Ma
> Ra Ma Da Sa
> Sa Sey So Hang

"The word *Kauri* means twenty & refers to the 20 sounds within the mantra. The first 7 sounds (**Sa Rey Ga Ma Pa Da Ni**) are known as *sargam*, (as in Sa-Re-Ga-Ma) or the Indian scale of music." For example, the comparative Western music scale is Do Re Mi Fa So La Ti Do. "The sargam is then followed by the *Panj Shabd*, then the *Siri Gaitri Mantra*. When the sargam & Panj Shabd are chanted together is it known as *Siri Sargam*."[90] (More information about Sa-Ta-Na-Ma on pg. 2. More information about Ra-Ma-Da-Sa-Sa-Sey-So-Hang on page 33).

"This is a mantra for the practice of Nada (Naad) Yoga in the Kundalini Yoga tradition. It balances the components of the earth and ether. When chanted in the Kriya format, it is of the essence of Saraswati, the Goddess of Nadam."[91]

KIRTAN SOHILA
Please see Kirtan Sohila Section (pg. 132)

LONG TIME SUN
Please see Frequently Used Kundalini Yoga Mantras (pg. 2)

MAAA
Divine Shield Meditation Mantra[92]

> Maaa, Maaa, Maaa

This is a mantra to the Universal Mother.

The sound 'Ma' represents the Mother throughout the world. It "calls on compassion and protection. Here, your soul is the child, and the universe becomes the Mother. If you call, She will come to your aid and comfort."[93]

MAHA MRITYUNJAI MANTRA
From Shukla-Yajur Veda - Waves of the Ganges Meditation Mantra[94]

Om Trayambakam Yajamahey
Sūgandin Pushtivardanam
Urva Rūkamiva Bandanan
Mrïtyor Mūkshia Mamritat

We worship the Supreme Light, the Three-Eyed One, Shiva, who is fragrant and sustains all beings
Just as the ripe cucumber is severed from the bondage of the vine, may we be delivered from the cycle of death and bestow upon us the nectar of life[95]

Om	= All that which is; the primal sound beyond the manifest realm
Trayambakam	= The Three-Eyed One, Shiva
Traya	= Three
Amba	= Eye
Yajamahey	= To sing Thy praise, worship
Sūgandin	= Fragrance
Pushtivardanam	= That which increases nourishment and prosperity
Pushti	= A well-nourished condition, prosperous
Vardanam	= One who strengthens health and well-being
UrvaRukamiva	= Deadly or overpowering disease
Urvarukam	= Cucumber
Iva	= Like
Urva	= Big and powerful, deadly
Arukam	= Disease
Bandanan	= Stem of a gourd; bound down, unhealthy attachment
Mrïtyor	= From death
Mūkshia	= Liberation
Mamritat	= Give us *Amrita* to be removed from the cycle of rebirth
Ma	= Give us
Amrita	= Nectar of Life

This mantra is The Great-Death Conquering Mantra. **Maha** means *great*; **Mrityos** means *of death*; **Jai** is *victory*[96]. It is a prayer for liberation from the repeating cycle of reincarnation and the suffering that must be endured throughout the resolution of our karmas. *Maha Mrityunjai Mantra* protects from disease and misfortunes as its vibration envelopes the body like a protective shield. This mantra is occasionally concluded with the word **Swaha** "which offers the enlightenment attained to God for all beings."[97] It is one of the only mantras that Yogi Bhajan ever shared that have a direct reference to **Shiva** and that contain the sacred Hindu sound 'Om'.

MANGALA SAJ BEYA
From Guru Arjun Dev Ji

Mangala Saj Beya Prab Ap-na Gai-a Ram
Abūnasi Var Sūni-a Man Up-ji-a Chai-a Ram
Man Prit Lagey Vadey Bagey Kab Mïli-ey Puran Patey
Sejey Samai-ey Govïnd Pai-ey Dey-o Saki-ey Mohe Matey
Dïn Reyn Tadi Kara-o Seyva Prab Kavan Jūgti Pai-a
Bïnvant Nanïk Karahu Kirpa Lehu Mohe Lar Lai-a

"The time of rejoicing has come; I sing of my Lord God. I have heard of my Imperishable Beloved Lord, and happiness fills my mind. My mind is in love with Him; when shall I realize my great fortune, and meet my Perfect Husband? If only I could meet the Lord of the Universe, and be automatically absorbed into Him; tell me how, O my companions! Day and night, I stand and serve my God; how can I attain Him? Nanak prays, have mercy on me, and attach me to the hem of Your robe, O Lord."[98]

This mantra is believed to connect one with her/his soul mate and to overcome lonliness.

ME WITHIN ME
Mantra Meditation for Self-Affirmation[99]

Me Within Me is the Purity
Me within Me Is The Reality
Me Within Me Is The Grace
I Am The Master Of The Space

MERE MAN LOCHEY
Verse 1 from Shabd Hazarey of Guru Arjun Dev Ji (pg. 63) - Meditation to Heal the Wounds of Love[100]

Aad Sach Jūgad Sach Hey BEY Sach Nanïk Hosi BEY Sach

Mere Man Lochey Gur Darshan Ta-I   Bïlap Karey Chatrik Ki Ni-a-I
Trika Na Utarey Sant Na Avey   Bïn Darshan Sant Pi-arey Jio
Ho Goli Jio Gol Gūma-I   Gur Darshan Sant Pi-arey Jio
Aad Sach Jūgad Sach Hey BEY Sach Nanïk Hosi BEY Sach

Teyra Mūk Suhava Ji-o Sahaj Dūn Bani Chir Ho-a Deykey Saring Pani
Dan So Deys Jaha Tu Vasi-a   Meyrey Sajan Mit Murarey Jio
Ho Goli Ho Gol Guma-I   Gur Sajan Mit Murarey Jio
Aad Sach Jūgad Sach Hey BEY Sach Nanïk Hosi BEY Sach

Ik Gari Na Milatey Ta Kalijūg Hota   Hūn Kad Mïli-ai Prai-a Tūd Bagavanta
Mo-eh Ren Na Vïhavey Nid Na Avey   Bïn Deykey Gur Darbarey Jio
Ho Goli Jio Gol Gūma-I   Tïs Sachey Gur Darbarey Jio

29

Aad Sach Jūgad Sach Hey BEY Sach Nanïk Hosi BEY Sach

Bag Ho-a Gur Sant Mïla-ia   Prab Abïnasi Gar Meh Pai-a
Seyv Kari Pal Chasa Na Vichura   Jan Nanïk Das Tūmarey Jio
Ho Goli Jio Gol Gūma-I   Jan Nanïk Das Tūmarey Jio
Aad Sach Jūgad Sach Hey BEY Sach Nanïk Hosi BEY Sach (4X)

"My mind longs for the Guru's Darshan (the sight of the Guru). It cries out like the thirsty song bird for the nectar of your name. My thirst is not quenched, and I can not find peace until I receive the Darshan of the beloved saint.

True in the beginning, True through all the ages, True even now, Nanak says Truth shall ever be. (Repeats after each verse, then repeats 4x at the end.)

I give myself, and my soul for your Darshan, my beloved Guru! Your face is so beautiful, and the sound of your words (shabd) is so filled with inner wisdom. It has been too long since this rain bird has had even a glimpse of water. Blessed is the land where you live, my friend and loved one, my Divine teacher.

I give myself, and my soul, to my beloved, my Divine Guru. An instant away from you, brings darkness. When will I meet You, my beloved Wahe Guru? I can't endure this night; sleep eludes me too. Until I see your home, my beloved Guru!

I give myself and my soul to your true home, my beloved Guru! By good fortune, I met my Saint Guru and I have found that the immortal creator is within the home of my own self and so I will always serve you and never be separated from you even for an instant. Guru Nanak says 'I'm your slave, my beloved Lord'. I give myself and my soul. Servant Nanak lives to serve you."[101]

This shabd was written as letters from Guru Arjun to his father Guru Ram Das.

"Whosoever will read these four letters shall become MY soul, MY projection, shall heal people, shall have places. Wealth will go after him again & again. There'll be nothing in the life of that man which he will fall short of."[102]

For Healing the Wounds of Love Meditation, this entire mantra is to be chanted 11 times each day for 11 days.

MUL MANTRA
Please see Aquarian Sadhana Mantras Section (pg. 3)

ON THIS DAY
The Kundalini Yoga Birthday Blessing - Words by Livtar Singh[103]

> On This Day The Lord Gave You Life, May You Use It To Serve Him (Her)
> All Of Our Loving Prayers Will Be With You, May You Never Forget Him (Her)
> May The Long Time Sun Shine Upon You, All Love Surround You
> And the Pure Light Within You, Guide Your Way On

ONG

Ong is the primal vibration from which all creativity flows. It is the creative manifestation of the infinite that we perceive through our senses. While *Om* is an ancient mantra of ascetics (yogis who left their homes and villages to live out life in isolation and deep practice), *Ong* is the mantra of the house-holder. The variation in the permutation of the sound applies to those yogis living modern lives; those holding jobs, raising families, driving cars and immersed in the culture of modernity. Chanting the sound **Ong** is done by using the back of the tongue to direct the air through the nasal sinus and out of the nostrils. This direction of the sound stimulates the pituitary gland, via the sphenoid, while vibrating the sutures that link the 8 cranial bones.

"**Ong Shabd** is the creative sound of the word *Om. Om* cannot be chanted, cannot be heard, cannot be sung, but you can create it. It is a creative word. That is why Guru Nanak used *Ong*. It is the right pronunciation of the word *Om. Ong* means creative force of God. It is created in the conch (nasal cavity), not with the mouth, not within, it is created in the conch of the human brain. The Sound *Ong* must be mastered. After mastering *Ong*, when you chant '*Ong Namo Guru Deyv Namo*', the Universe will open up to you."[104]

ONG KAR NIRANKAR

Ong Kar Nirankar Nirankar Ong

Ong Kar	= God in the Manifest Creation
Nirankar	= Formless God

ONG NAMO GURU DEYV NAMO
Adi Mantra - I bow to the Divine Wisdom & Divine Teacher that is within My Self
Please see Frequently Used Kundalini Yoga Mantras (pg. 1)

ONG SOHANG

Ong is the creative manifestation of the infinite that we perceive through our senses
Sohang means *I am Thou*

Chanting **Ong** enhances our perception of time/space and deeply affects the Pituitary Gland. The sound **Hang** (pronounced like '*hung*') "stimulates and opens Anahata Chakra (Heart)"[105].

PARAMEYSAREY
From Guru Arjun Dev Ji

Aad Puran	= In the beginning, pervading, perfect
Mad Puran	= In the middle, pervading, perfect
Aant Puran	= In the end, pervading, perfect
Parmeysarey	= Transcendent Lord Master
Parmeysarey Dita Bana	= The Transcendent Lord has given me his Support
Dūk Rog Ka Deyra Bana	= The house of pain and disease has been destroyed
Aanad Kareh Nar Nari	= Men and Women celebrate in bliss
Har Har Prab Kirpa Dari	= The Lord God, Har, Har has extended mercy

The first four lines of this mantra are in *Rag Sorath* and the last four are in *Rag Jaithsri*.

PAVAN GURU
Pran Bhanda Meditation Mantra[106]

Pavan Pavan Pavan Pavan
Par Para Pavan Guru
Pavan Guru Wahe Guru
Wahe Guru Pavan Guru

May the breath of life remove from you any darkness that you may have a glimpse of ecstasy

Pavan	= Air of the breath
Guru	= Teacher, wisdom
Wahe	= WOW
Gu	= Darkness, stickiness
Ru	= Remover of

"This mantra forges a link between you as a finite unit magnetic field and the universal, creative magnetic field of energy that we call consciousness. One who practices this to perfection experiences deathlessness. This meditation can give you the capacity to embody a divine personality, and to become creative and fearless."[107]

Wahe Guru = Great Beyond Description is the experience of God's Infinite Wisdom
Pavan is air, the vehicle through which prana (life force) enters our being
Pavan Guru is the divine wisdom that flows through the breath
Waheguru is also a term used in modern Punjabi that is synonymous with *God*

PEOPLE OF LOVE
Words by Yogi Bhajan & Snatam Kaur[108]

Chorus:
We are the People the People of Love Let us People Love today

We are one under the sun let your heart sing it this way
Love is something as free as the wind I say it to you and I say it again

Reach out to the one you don't know and give him a helping hand
The time has come for our sacrifice to find the way to our Love

PRANA APANA SUSHUMNA

Prana Apana Sushumna Hari, Hari Har Hari Har Hari Har Hari

Prana = The Vayu (*wind*) that moves from the heart to the neck. It is linked to the function of the lungs and to inspiration.
Apana = The Vayu below the naval that is associated with elimination through the rectum, the bladder, the colon and the genitals.
Sushumna = The central channel and primary nadi through which Kundalini flows upward as a result of the union of prana flowing from Ida & Pingala Nadis.[109]

Har	= Creative Infinite aspect of God
Hari	= Creation in Action

Sushumna is the primary **nadi**, or channel through which energy flows in the body. **Ida** is the feminine, receptive channel of energy that begins at the base of the torso (*muladhara chakra*) and spirals up to the left nostril (*ajna chakra*). **Pingala** is the masculine channel of energy that begins at the base of the torso (*muladhara chakra*) and spirals up to the right nostril (*ajna chakra*). **Ida** & **Pingala** intersect with each of the major chakras and meet where *Sushumna* begins.[110]

RA MA DA SA
Siri Gaitri Mantra for Healing[111]

Ra Ma Da Sa		Sa Sey So Hang	
Ra	= Sun	**Sa**	= Impersonal Infinity
Ma	= Moon	**Sey**	= Thou
Da	= Earth	**So**	= Personal sense of merger & identity
Sa	= Impersonal Infinity	**Hang**	= The Infinite, Vibrating & Real
Sa+Say = Totality of Infinity		**So+Hang** = "I Am Thou"	

This mantra is a healing mantra in Kundalini Yoga and is an attunement of the self to the universe. These eight sounds stimulate the Kundalini flow in the central channel of the spine for healing. *Hang* rhymes with the English word *rung*.

RA MA

Raa Maa   or   Raa Raa Raa Raa Maa Maa Maa Maa

Ra = Sun, Male   Ma = Moon, Female

Chanting this mantra brings balance of the male and female aspects in the psyche.

RA RA RA RA MA MA MA MA

Ra Ra Ra Ra, Ma Ma Ma Ma, Sa Sa Sa Sat, Hari Har Hari Har[112]

or

Ra Ra Ra Ra, Ma Ma Ma Ma, Rama Rama Rama Ram, Sa Ta Na Ma[113]

Ra	= Sun, Male	Har	= Creative Infinite aspect of God
Ma	= Moon, Female	Sa	= Infinity, cosmos, beginning
Sa	= Impersonal Infinity	Ta	= Life, existence
Sat	= Truth	Na	= Death, change, transformation
Hari	= Creation in Action	Ma	= Rebirth

This mantra balances the male/female aspects of the self, the hemispheres of the brain, and the sense of identity.

RAK-E RAKANA HAR
Final Verse from Rehiras Sahib of Guru Arjun Dev Ji (pg. 123)
Please see Aquarian Sadhana Mantras Section (pg. 4)

RAM RAM HARI RAM

Ram Ram Hari Ram

Ram = 7th incarnation of Vishnu; he took birth to free the world of cruelty & sins
Hari = Creation in Action

"The first *Ram* invokes creativity and blessing of the universal magnetic field and existence. The second *Ram* consolidates and protects that magnetic field and creation. The third *Ram* completes and gives peace through the time of death. The final *Hari's* are the platform of the four corners that elevate you in consciousness as you journey across earth."[114]

"The first half of the mantra is a relationship in *Nad* (Naad or Nadam) to the infinite and formless existence and nonexistence. The second half is guidance through the experiences of form and earth. Together the two parts of this mantra are a polarity that takes you beyond polarity to experience and project your original self."[115]

Ram is commonly used as a sound for God.

RERIHAS SAHIB
Please see Rehiras Sahib Section (pg. 114)

REY MAN SHABD
From Guru Gobind Singh

Rey Man-eh Bïd Jog Kama-o
Sïngi Sach Akapat Kantala
Di-an Bibūt Chara-o
Tati Gaho Atam Bas Kar Ki
Bicha Nam Aad-arang
Bajey Param Tar Tat Har Ko
Upajey Rag Ras-arang
Ugatey Tan Tarang Rang
At Gi-an Git Band-anang
Chak Chak Rehey Deyv Danav Mūn
Chak Chak Beyom Biv-anang
Atam Upadeys Beys Sanjam Ko
Jap So Ajapa Japey
Sada Reyhey Kanchan Si Kaya
Kal Na Kabahū Beyapey

"Oh my mind, practice yoga in this way:
Let truth be your horn, sincerity your necklace and Meditation the ashes you apply on your body. Catch your burning soul and stop the flames. Let the soul be the bowl that you collect Nam with. This will be the only support you will ever need. The universe plays its divine music. The sound of reality is shrill, but this is where God is. When you listen to the reality from this place of awareness the sweet essence of Rag arises. Waves of melodies, emotions and passions arise and flow through you. Bind yourself with the song of God. The universe spins like a potter's wheel and from it fly demons and angels. The sage listens to this, and instead of getting caught in either one, drinks from the nectar of the heavens and is carried there in a divine chariot. Instruct and clothe yourself with self-control. Meditate unto infinity until you are meditating without meditating. In this way, your body shall remain forever golden and death shall never approach you."[116]

This mantra is a poem by *Guru Gobind Singh*, the 10th Master of the Sikh lineage. It basically describes the way to practice yoga. This mantra is said to be a powerful way to augment one's yoga practice. According Mahan Kirn Kaur, this particular mantra is an excellent way to deepen the experience of consciousness while practicing Bound Lotus Kriya.[117]

35

SA REY SA SA
Antar Nad Mudra Mantra (Kabadshe Meditation Mantra)[118]

Sa Rey Sa Sa	Har Rey Har Har
Sa Rey Sa Sa	Har Rey Har Har
Sa Rey Sa Sa	Har Rey Har Har
Sa Rang	Har Rang

"*Sa* is the Infinite, the Totality, God. It is the element of ether. *Har* is the creativity of the Earth. It is dense; the power of manifestation. These sounds are woven together & projected through the sound of *Ang,* (rhymes with *sung*) or complete Totality. It gives you the capacity of effective communication so your words contain mastery & impact. *Antar Nad Mudra* is the meditation that opens the chakras for the full effect of any other mantra."[119]

SATGURU HO-EY DYAL
By Guru Arjun Dev Ji

Satïgur Ho-ey Deyal Ta Sarda Pori-ey	= Your trust is complete
Satïgur Ho-ey Deyal Na Kabahū Jūri-ey	= You will never turn away in grief
Satïgur Ho-ey Deyal Ta Dūk Na Jani-ey	= You will not know suffering
Satïgur Ho-ey Deyal Ta Har Ran Mani-ey	= You will enjoy God's Love
Satïgur Ho-ey Deyal Ta Jam Kar Dar Key-a	= What reason is there to fear death
Satïgur Ho-ey Deyal Ta Sad Hi Sūk Dey-a	= The body is ever in peace
Satïgur Ho-ey Deyal Ta Nad Nïd Pai-ey	= The 9 treasures come to you
Satïgur Ho-ey Deyal Ta Sach Samai-ey	= Then you are absorbed in truth

The opening words of each line, **Satïgur Ho-ey Deyal**, mean *"The True Guru is merciful"*.

SAT KARTAR
God, the Doer of Truth

Sat	= Truth
Kartar	= The 'Doer' aspect of God

"*Sat Kartar* is a sound that Guru Nanak, founder of the Sikh Path, (from which many Kundalini Yoga mantras have come) would speak when things would happen, good or bad. His response was, '*Sat Kartar!*' and in effect he was saying, '*God or the Great Divine One, is the One doing this action, this situation*'. The *Sat* in the mantra is first identifying the Soul's True Sound, *Essence of Truth, or Being...* it is a key to living in a state of faith."[120]

SAT NAM
Please see Frequently Used Kundalini Yoga Mantras (pg. 2)

SAT NAM WAHE GURU
2010 3HO Global Meditation: Fire Tatva – Fire Kriya Mantra[121]

> Sat Nam Sat Nam Sat Nam Sat Nam
> Sat Nam Sat Nam Wahe Guru

When rhythmically chanted in the kriya format, "this mantra develops will power and gives the capacity to understand the elements of your personality. It is perfect to overcome difficulty in completing projects and doing what you intend."[122]

This mantra is also found within other kriyas such as *Tapa Yog Karam Kriya*[123].

SAT NARAYAN
2009 3HO Global Meditation: Water Tatva - Narayan Kriya Mantra[124] *(Chotay Pad Mantra)*

> Sat Narayan Wahe Guru
> Hari Narayan Sat Nam

or

> Sat Narayan Hari Narayan
> Hari Narayan Hari Hari

Sat Narayan	= The True Sustainer
Wahe Guru	= Indescribable Wisdom
Hari	= Creation in Action
Sat Nam	= True identity
Nara	= Water (Sanskrit)
Ayana	= Resting place of Lord Vishnu

"Chanting this mantra makes you intuitively clear and pure in your consciousness. Even a person with low self-esteem can become majestic by chanting it. The words invoke the various names of God to help bring prosperity, peace of mind, and the capacity to look beyond this world to realize the Infinite."[125]

Chotay Pad literally means *small step.*
Narayan is a form of the God *Vishnu* and is representative of the water element.

SAT SIRI SIRI AKAL
Please see Aquarian Sadhana Mantras Section (pg. 4)

SHABD HAZAREY
Please see Shabd Hazarey Section (pg. 63)

SO PURKH
Verse From Rehiras Sahib of Guru Ram Das (pg. 116)

Rag Asa Mehla Chauta So Purk
Ek Ong Kar Satïgur Prasad
So Purk Niranjan Har Purk
Niranjan Har Agma Agam Apara
Sab Di-ave Sab Di-ave
Tūd Ji Har Sachey Sirjan-hara
Sab Ji-a Tūmarey
Ji Tu Ji-a Ka Datara
Har Di-avahu Santahu
Ji Sab Dūk Visaran-hara
Har Apey Takur Har Apey
Seyvek Ji Ki-a Nanïk Jant Vichara
Tu Gat Gat Antar Sarab Nirantar
Ji Har Eyko Purk Samana
Ek Datey-ek Bey-kari
Ji Sab Teyrey Choj Vidana

Tu Apey Data Apey Bhūgta
Ji Ha-o Tūdh Bïn Avar Na Jana
Tu Par-brahm Bey-ant Bey-ant
Ji Teyrey Ki-a Gūn Aak Vakana
Jo Seyveh Jo Seyveh Tūd Ji
Jan Nanïk Tïn Kūbana
Har Di-avahe Har Di-avahe
Tūd Ji Sey Jan Jūg Meh Sūkvasi

Sey Mūkat Sey Mūkat Ba-ey Jïn Har
Dia-ia Ji Tïn Tūti Jam Ki Fasi
Jïn Nirbao Jïn Har Nirbao Dia-ia
Ji Tïn Ka Ba-o Sab Gavasi
Jïn Seyvi-a Jïn Seyvi-a Meyra
Har Ji Tey Har Har Rūp Samasi
Sey Dan Sey Dan Jïn Har Dia-ia
Ji Jan Nanïk Tïn Bal Jasi

Teyri Bagat Teyri Bagat Bandar
Ji Barey Bi-ant Bey-anta
Teyrey Bagat Teyrey Bagat Salahan
Tūd Ji Har Anek Aneyk Ananta
Teyri Anek Teyri Anek Karahi Har
Pūja Ji Tap Tapeh Japeh Bey-anta
Teyrey Anek Teyrey Anek Pareh Baho Sïmrat Sasat
Ji Kar Kïri-a Kat Karam Karanta

Sey Bagat Sey Bagat Baley Jan Nanïk
Ji Jo Baveh Meyrey Har Bagvanta

Tu Aad Purk Aprampar Karta
Ji Tūd Jeyvad Avar Na Ko-i
Tu Jūg Jūg Eyko Sada Sada Tu Eyko
Ji Tu Nehechal Karta So-i
Tūd Apey Bavey So-i Vartey
Ji Tu Apey Karahi So Ho-i
Tūd Apey Sarïst Sab Upa-i
Ji Tūd Apey Siraj Sab Go-i

Jan Nanïk Gūn Gavey Kartey
Key Ji Jo Sab-sey Ka Jano-i

That Primal Being is Immaculate and Pure. The Lord, the Primal Being, is Immaculate and Pure. The Lord is Unrivalled. All meditate; all meditate on You, Dear Lord, O True Creator Lord. All living beings are Yours; You are the Giver of all souls. Meditate on the Lord, O Saints; He is the Dispeller of all sorrow. The Lord Himself is the Master; the Lord Himself is the Servant. O Nanak, the poor beings are wretched and miserable!

You are constant in each and every heart, and in all things. O Dear Lord, you are the One. Some are givers, and some are beggars. This is all Your Wondrous Play. You Yourself are the Giver, and You Yourself are the Enjoyer. I know no other than You. You are the Supreme Lord God, Limitless and Infinite. What Virtues of Yours can I speak of and describe? Unto those who serve You, unto those who serve You, Dear Lord, servant Nanak is a sacrifice.

Those who meditate on You, Lord; those who meditate on You; those humble beings dwell in peace in this world. They are liberated; they are liberated, those who meditate on the Lord. For them, the noose of death is cut away. Those who meditate on the Fearless One, on the Fearless Lord - all their fears are dispelled. Those who serve; those who serve my Dear Lord, are absorbed into the Being of the Lord, Har, Har. Blessed are they; blessed are they, who meditate on their Dear Lord. Servant Nanak is a sacrifice to them.

Devotion to You; devotion to You, is a treasure overflowing, infinite and beyond measure. Your devotees; Your devotees praise You, Dear Lord, in many and various and countless ways. For You, many; for You, so very many perform worship services, O Dear Infinite Lord; they practice disciplined meditation and chant endlessly. For You, many; for You, so very many read the various Simritees and Shastras. They perform rituals and religious rites. Those devotees; those devotees are sublime, O servant Nanak, who are pleasing to my Dear Lord God.

You are the Primal Being, the Most Wonderful Creator. There is no other as Great as You. Age after age; You are the One. Forever & ever, You are the One. You never change, O Creator Lord. Everything happens according to Your Will. You Yourself accomplish all that occurs. You Yourself created the entire universe, and having fashioned it, You shall destroy it all. Servant Nanak sings the Glorious Praises of the Dear Creator, the Knower of all.[126]

39

"This Mantra creates a sacred space in which grace prevails so as to allow the greatness of the soul to come forth. It was written by Guru Ram Das, whose vibrations hold a great state of love that heals all realms of the heart and being. Yogi Bhajan said if a woman recites this Bani (sacred hymn) 11 times a day for any man, it has the power to make him a saint and to dissolve any negativity existing between them."[127]

So Purkh is a part of *Rehiras*, the evening prayer of the Sikhs. It is said that a woman can recite this to bring a man into her life or to give help to a man she is already with.

SOCHEY SOCH
Please see Japji Sahib, 1ˢᵗ Pauri (pg. 44-Transliteration & pg. 53-Translation)

SOI SUNANDARI
From Guru Arjun Dev Ji

So-i Sūnandari Mera Tan Man Mola = Hearing of Thee my body and mind blossom
Nam Japandari Lali = I contemplate the Name of my Beloved
Pand Jūlandari Mera Andar Tanda = Walking your path my inner being is cooled
Guru-darshan Deyk Nihali = Seeing your vision, I am blessed

This mantra is to invoke the presence and protection of Guru Ram Das, who is the father of Guru Arjun Dev Ji.

SVAYE
Please see Tav Prasad Svaye Section (pg. 98)

SUNI-EY
Please Japji Sahib, 8ᵗʰ – 11ᵗʰ Pauri (pg. 45-Transliteration & pg. 54-Translation)

TAV PRASAD SVAYE
Please see Tav Prasad Svaye Section (pg. 98)

TERI MEHR DA BOLNA

Teri Mer Da Bolna   Aad Gurey Nameh
Tūd Agey Ardas   Jūgad Gurey Nameh
Guru Guru Wahe Guru   Sat Gurey Nameh
Guru Ram Das   Sïri Guru Deyv-ey Nameh

"Oh Guru Ram Das, this is my prayer to you. May my words be from you and may my mind be a source of knowledge and ecstasy that wisdom may come as I act as a servant of the Infinite. I bow to the primal wisdom; I bow to the wisdom true through the ages; I bow to the true wisdom; I bow to the great unseen wisdom."[128]

"He (Yogi Bhajan) always said that every thing that he taught came from the grace of Guru Ram Das. Before every lecture he chanted this mantra."[129]

TRIPLE MANTRA[130]
Mangalacharn Mantra with Kundalini Shakti Mantra

Aad Gurey Nameh	= I bow to the primal wisdom
Jūgad Gurey Nameh	= I bow to the wisdom true through the ages
Sat Gurey Nameh	= I bow to the true wisdom
Sïri Guru Deyv-ey Nameh	= I bow to the great unseen wisdom
Aad Sach	= True in the beginning
Jūgad Sach	= True through all the ages
Hey Bi Sach	= True even now
Nanïk Hosi BI Sach	= Nanak says Truth shall ever be
Aad Sach	= True in the beginning
Jūgad Sach	= True through all the ages
Hey Bi Sach	= True even now
Nanïk Hosi BEY Sach	= Nanak says Truth shall ever be

"When you cannot be protected, this mantra shall protect you. When things stop and won't move, this makes them move in your direction."[131]

Triple Mantra helps clear all types of mental, psychic and physical obstacles in one's daily life. It cuts through opposing vibrations, thoughts, words and actions. Triple Mantra is said to protect one from car, plane or automobile accidents.[132]

WAH YANTI
Please see Aquarian Sadhana Mantras Section (pg. 3)

WAHE GURU
2012 3HO Global Meditation: Ether Tatva Meditation Mantra[133]

Wahe = WOW, ecstasy		**Guru** = Teacher, wisdom	
Gu = Darkness, stickiness		**Ru** = Remover of	

Great Beyond Description is the experience of God's Infinite Wisdom

It is commonly said by teachers of Kundalini Yoga that chanting 'Wahe Guru' once is as powerful as chanting Har 1,000 times. It is the mantra of ecstasy. In modern Punjabi, *Waheguru* has become a term synonomous with 'God'.

"If you say, *Har* 1100 times, and you correctly say, *Wa-Hey Guru* once... everything has a little bit of speciality about it".[134]

WAHE GURU WAHE JIO
Please see Aquarian Sadhana Mantras Section (pg. 5)

WA WA HEY HEY
Nad Meditation Mantra: To Communicate from Totality[135]

Wa Wa Hey Hey, Wa Wa Hey Hey, Wa Wa Hey Hey Gu Ru

Wahe = WOW, ecstasy	**Guru** = Teacher, wisdom
Gu = Darkness, stickiness	**Ru** = Remover of

When done in the Nad (*naad*) Meditation form, "this mantra allows one to merge into the feeling of totality. When one speaks from that feeling of totality, trust is created. With trust, strong relationships are established."[136]

WE ARE PEACE
Words by Yogi Bhajan, Snatam Kaur & Jeffrey Armstrong[137]

Chorus:
We are light, We are love, We are peace

I feel your love
Calling out to me
In the rhythm of your heart
A journey to be free
Carried by the One
Hand in hand we'll go
You are so beautiful
So let your spirit flow

Chorus

In the warmth of the sun
In the cool of the moon
I feel it in my soul
And I know that it's true
In the bliss of love
A smile upon your face
The light of children and giving
Fills the world with grace

Bridge:
May peace prevail
May mankind live in absolute joy
Happiness and prosperity
And may we understand each other
In trust and affection

SACRED NITNEM

The 7 Banis, or sacred hymns, featured in this section contain the obligatory prayers to be recited daily by practicing Sikhs. These Banis were originally given by the Satgurus of the the Sikh lineage. With the exception of Japji Sahib, these hymns in their entirety do not have a direct relationship to Kundalini Yoga as it is most commonly taught; however, Yogi Bhajan made reference to them frequently during his many years of teaching. To omit them would be to omit gems of timeless beauty and grace.

The word *nitnem* is a compound word meaning **daily observance**.

Nït = Daily, continual
Nem = Practice, rule, regimen[138]

"There are two words which can decide the entire categorization of this Dharma: **Nitnem** & Nimet. **Nitnem,** (means) daily. Nimita, (means) for the sake of. If Sikh lives for the sake of the Guru, God serves such a Sikh."[139]

The transliterations and translations are each presented in their entirety for greater ease in following along in the Aquarian Sadhana experience. Immerse and enjoy!

JAPJI SAHIB OF GURU NANAK DEV JI

The Kundalini Yoga Aquarian Sadhana practice begins with this prayer, *Japji Sahib*. Read in its' entirety it can take between 15 and 25 minutes, depending upon the familiarity and intention of the reader. This *bani*, or prayer, is begun at the hour of 4 A.M. It is composed of 38 *pauris*, or stanzas, plus the final sermon called the *slok*.

Guru Nanak Dev Ji was the First Guru and the founder of the Sikh lineage. It is widely believed that he was born April 15, 1469 in what is currently Pakistan. The birthday (*jayanti*) of Guru Nanak falls on Kartik Purnima, the day of the full moon in the month of Kartik. In the Gregorian calendar, the birthday of Guru Nanak usually falls in the month of November, but its date varies from year to year, based on the traditional dates of the Indian calendar,[140] which is a lunar system. It is a national holiday in India.

The story of the first part of *Japji Sahib*, called the *Mul Mantra* (root mantra) has been told and retold. Here is one version of the story:

Guru Nanak spent much of his time practicing his *sadhana*, or daily practice. It is said that part of his practice was done by purifying himself in the river, next to which he meditated. One day, upon immersing himself, he disappeared beneath the waters surface for three days. Upon his emergence he is said to have had a glowing light surrounding him that was so pronounced, even those who were not disposed to seeing auras noticed. In his exalted state of awareness, he spoke the words of the *Mul Mantra* in order to communicate to the surrounding students the enraptured state of being he had experienced.[141]

Each *pauri*, or stanza, in this powerful expression of the Sacred Sound Current (*Shabd Guru*) contains a gem of wisdom. According to Yogi Bhajan, each *pauri* works a different facet necessary for soul activation. Those effects, from the teachings of Yogi Bhajan[142], are listed beneath each translation[143] *in italics* (below the transliteration section).

Japji Sahïb

Ek ong kar sat nam
Karta purk nirbhao nir-ver
Akal mūrït ajūni
Saibang gūr prasad Jap!
Aad sach jūgad sach heybi sach
Nanïk hosi bi sach ||1||

Sochey soch na hovi jey sochi lak var
Chūpey chūp na hovi jey lai raha lïv tar
Būki-a būk na ūtri jey bana puri-a bar
Sehas si-anpa lak ho-e ta ïk na chaley nal
Kiv sachi-ara ho-i-ey kiv kūrey tūtey pal
Hūkam raja-i chalna Nanïk lïki-a nal ||1||

Hūkmi hovan akar hūkam na kahi-a ja-i
Hūkmi hovan ji-a hūkam mïley vadia-i
Hūkmi ūtam nich hūkam lïk dūk sūk pai-ey
Ïkna hūkmi baksis ïk hūkmi sada bavai-ey
Hūkmey andar sab ko bahar hūkam na ko-i
Nanïk hūkmey jey būjey ta hūmeu kahey na ko-I ||2||

Gavai ko tan hovey kïsey tan
Gavai ko dat janey ni-san
Gavai ko gūn vadia-ia char
Gavai ko vïdi-a vikam vichar
Gavai ko saj karey tan key
Gavai ko ji-a ley fïr dey
Gavai ko japey disey dor
Gavai ko vey-key hadra hador
Kat-na kati na avey tot
Kat kat kati koti kot kot
Deyda dey ley-dey tak pai
Jūga jūgantar ka-i kai
Hūkmi hūkam chala-ey ra
Nanïk vig-sey vey-parvau ||3||

Sacha sa-ib sach na-i baki-a ba-o apar
Akey man-gey dey-i dey-i dat karey datar
Feyr ki agey raki-ey jït dïsai dar-bar
Muho ki bolan boli-ey jït sūn darey pi-ar
Amrit veyla sach na-o vadi-a-i vichar
Karmi avey kapra nadri mok du-ar
Nanïk ey-vey jani-ey sab apey sachi-ar ||4||

44

Tapi-a na ja-i kita na ho-i
Apey aap niranjan so-i
Jïn seyvi-a tïn pa-i-a man
Nanïk gavi-ey gūni nidan
Gavi-ey sūni-ey man raki-ey bao
Dūk par-har sūk gar ley ja-i
Gurmūk nadang gurmūk veydang gurmūk reyhia sama-i
Gur isar gur gork barma gur parbati ma-i
Jey hao jana aka na-i keh-na katan na ja-i
Gura ïk deyi būja-I sabna ji-a ka ïk data so mey vïsar na ja-i ||5||

Tirat nava jey tïs bava vïn baney ki na-i kari
Jeyti sirat ūpa-i veyka vïn karma ki mïley la-i
Mat vïch ratan javahar manïk jey ïk gur ki sïk sūni
Gura ïk dey-i būja-i sabna ji-a ka ïk data so mey visar na ja-i ||6||

Jey jūg charey arja hor dasūni ho-i
Nava kanda vïch jani-ey nal chaley sab ko-i
Changa na-o raka-i key jas kirat jag ley-i
Jey tïs nadar na avi ta vat na pūchey key
Kita andar kit kar dosi dos darey
Nanïk nirgūn gūn karey gūnvan-ti-a gūn dey
Teyha ko-i na sūja-i jï tïs gūn ko-i karey ||7||

Sūni-ey sïd pir sur nat
Sūni-ey darat daval akas
Sūni-ey dip lo-a patal
Sūni-ey pohi na sakey kal
Nanïk bag-ta sada vigas
Sūni-ey dūk pap ka nas ||8||

Sūni-ey isar barma ïnd
Sūni-ey mūk salahan mand
Sūni-ey jog jūgat tan beyd
Sūni-ey sasat sïmrït veyd
Nanïk bagta sada vigas
Sūni-ey dūk pap ka nas ||9||

Sūni-ey sat santok gi-an
Sūni-ey at-sat ka isnan
Sūni-ey par par paveh man
Sūni-ey lagey sahaj di-an
Nanïk bagta sada vigas
Sūni-ey dūk pap ka nas ||10||

Sūni-ey sara gūna key ga
Sūni-ey seyk pir pat-sa

Sūni-ey andey paveh ra
Sūni-ey hat hovey asga
Nanïk bagta sada vigas
Sūni-ey dūk pap ka nas ||11||

Maney ki-gat ke-hi na ja-i
Jey ko kahey pïch-ey pach-utai
Kagad kalam na lïkan-har
Maney ka bey karan vichar
Eysa nam niranjan ho-i
Jey ko man janey man ko-i ||12||

Maney surat hovey man būd
Maney sagal bavan ki sūd
Maney mū chota na ka-i
Maney jam key sat na ja-i
Eysa nam niranjan ho-i
Jey ko man janey man ko-i ||13||

Maney mar-ag tak na pa-i
Maney pat si-o pargat ja-i
Maney mag na chaley pant
Maney daram sey-ti san-band
Eysa nam niranjan ho-i
Jey ko man janey man ko-i ||14||

Maney paveh mok duar
Maney parva-rey sadar
Maney tarey tareh gur sïk
Maney Nanïk bavey na bïk
Eysa nam niranjan ho-i
Jey ko man janey man ko-i ||15||

Panch parvan panch pardan
Panchey paveh dargeh man
Panchey so-eh dar rajan
Pancha ka gur eyk dian
Jey ko kahey karey vichar
Kartey key karney nahi sūmar
Dūl Daram di-a ka pūt
Santok tap raki-a jïn sūt
Jey ko būjey hovey sachi-ar
Dav-ley ūpar keyta bar
Darti hor parey hor hor
Tis tey bar taley kavan jor
Ji-a jat ranga key nav
Sabna lïki-a vuri kalam
Eh leyka lïk janey ko-e
Leyka lïki-a keyta ho-e

Keyta tan su-ali rūp
Keyti dat janey kaun kūt
Kita pasa-o eyko kava-o
Tis tey ho-ey lak dari-ao
Kūdrat kavan kaha vichar
Vari-a na java eyk var
Jo tūd bavey sa-i bali kar
Tū sada salamat nirankar ||16||

Asank jap asank ba-o
Asank pūja asank tap ta-o
Asank grant mūk veyd path
Asank jog man ra-hey udas
Asank bagat gūn gi-an vichar
Asank sati asank datar
Asank sūr mū bak sar
Asank mon līv la-e tar
Kūdrat kavan kaha vichar
Vari-a na java eyk var
Jo tūd bavey sa-i bali kar
Tū sada salamat nirankar ||17||

Asank mūrak and gor
Asank chor haram-kor
Asank amar kar ja-eh jor.
Asank gal-vad hati-a kama-i
Asank papi pap kar ja-i.
Asank kūri-ar kūr-ey fira-i
Asank maleych mal bak ka-i
Asank nïn-dak sir kareh bar
Nanïk nich kahey vichar
Vari-a na java eyk var
Jo tūd bavey sa-i bali kar
Tū sada salamat nirankar ||18||

Asank nav asank tav
Agam agam asank lo-a
Asank kahey sir bar ho-e
Akri nam akri sala
Akri gi-an git gūn ga
Akri lïkan bolan ban
Akra sir sanjog vakan
Jïn-eh lïkey tïs sir na-i
Jïv furma-ey tïv tïv pa-i
Jeyta kita teyta na-o
Vïn navey na-i ko ta-o
Kūdrat kavan kaha vichar
Vari-a na java eyk var

Jo tūd bavey sa-i bali kar
Tū sada salamat nirankar ||19||

Bari-ey hat peyr tan dey
Pani dotey ūtras key
Mūt paliti kapar ho-e
Dey sabūn lai-ey oh Do-e
Bari-ey mat papa key sang
O Dopey navey key rang
Pūni papi akan na-i
Kar kar karna lïk ley ja-e
Apey bij apey hi ka-e
Nanïk hūkmi ava ja-e ||20||

Tirat tap dai-a dat dan
Jey ko pavey til ka man
Sūni-a mani-a man kita ba-o
Antargat tirat mal na-o
Sab gūn tey-rey mey na-i ko-i
Vïn gūn ki-tey bagat na ho-i
Su-ast at bani barma-o
Sat suhan sada man cha-o
Kavan su veyla vakat kavan kavan tït kavan var
Kavan si rūti ma kavan jït ho-a akar
Veyl na pai-a pand-ti ji hovey leyk puran
Vakat na pai-o kadi-a ji lïkan leyk kuran
Tït var na jogi janey rūt ma na ko-i
Ja karta sirti ko sajey apey janey so-i
Kiv kar aka kïv sala-i ki-o varni kïv jana
Nanïk akan sab ko akey ïk dū ïk si-ana
Vada sa-ib vadi nai kita ja ka hovey
Nanïk jey ko apo janey agey gai-a na sohey ||21||

Patala patal lak agasa agas
Ork Ork bal takey veyd kahan ïk vat
Sehas atara kahan kateyba asūlū ïk dat
Leyka hoi ta lïki-ey ley-key ho-i vinas
Nanïk vada aki-ey apey janey ap ||22||

Salahi salahi eyti surat na pai-a
Nadi-a atey va paveh samūnd na jani-ey
Samund sa sūltan gira seyti mal dan
Kiri tūl na hovni jey tïs mano na visa-rey ||23||

Ant-na sïfti kehan na-ant
Ant-na karney deyn na-ant
Ant-na veykan sūnan na-ant
Ant-na japey ki-a man mant
Ant-na japey kita akar

Ant-na japey paravar
Ant-ka ran key-tey bil lay
Ta key ant na pa-ey jai
Ey ant na janey ko-i
Bauta kai-ey bauta ho-i
Vada sa-ib ūcha ta-o
ūchey ūpar ūcha na-o
Eyvad ūcha hovey ko-i
Tïs ūchey kao janey so-i
Jey-vad aap janey aap aap
Nanïk nadri karmi dat ||24||

Ba-ota karam lïki-a na ja-i
Vada data tïl na tama-i
Key-tey man-gey jod apar
Keyti-a ganat na-i vichar
Key-tey kap tu-tey vey-kar
Key-tey ley ley mukar pa-i
Key-tey mūrk kahi ka-e
Keyti-a dūk būk sad mar
Ey-bi dat teyri datar
Band kalasi baney ho-i
Hor ak na sakey ko-i
Jey ko ka-ik akan pa-i
Oh janey jeyti-a mu ka-i
Apey janey apey de
Akey se bi key-i ke
Jïs no bak-sey sïfat sala
Nanïk pat-sahi pat-sa ||25||

Amūl gūn amūl vapar
Amūl vapari-ey amūl bandar
Amūl avey amūl ley jai
Amūl ba-i amūla samai
Amūl daram amūl diban
Amūl tūl amūl parvan
Amūl baksis amūl nisan
Amūl karam amūl fūr-man
Amūlo amūl akhi-a na ja-i
Aak aak rahey lïv la-i
Akey veyd pat pūran
Akey pa-rey ka-rey vaki-an
Akey bar-mey akey ind
Akey gopi tey govïnd
Akey isar akey sïd
Akey key-tey ki-tey būd
Akey danav akey deyv
Akey sūr nar mūn jan seyv

49

Key-tey akey akan pa-i
Key-tey key key ūt ūt ja-i
Ey-tey ki-tey hor kar-eh
Ta aak na sa-key key-i keh
Jey-vad bavey tey-vad ho-eh
Nanïk janey sacha so-eh
Jey ko akey bol-ïvïgar
Ta lïki-ey sir gavara gavar ||26||

So dar keyha so gar keyha jït bey sarab samaley
Vajey nad aneyk asanka key-tey vavan-harey
Key-tey rag pari si-o kehi-an key-tey gavan-harey
Gavey tūno paun pani beysantar gavey raja daram du-arey
Gavey chït gūpat lïk janey lïk lïk daram vicharey
Gavey isar bar-ma deyvi sohan sada savarey
Gavey ind indasan bey-tey deyva-ti-a dar naley
Gavey sïd samadi andar gavan sad vicharey
Gavey jati sati santoki gavey vir kararey
Gavan pandit parhan rakisar jūg jūg veyda naley
Gavey moni-a man mohan surga mach pia-ley
Gavan ratan upa-ey tey-rey atsat tirat naley
Gaveh jod mahabal sūra gavey kani charey
Gaveh kand mandal varbanda kar kar rakey darey
Sey tūd-no gaveh jo tūd bavan ratey tey-rey bagat rasaley
Hor key-tey gavan sey mey chit na avan Nanïk ki-a vicharey
So-i so-i sada sach sa-ib sacha sachi na-i
Hey bi hosi jai na jasi rachna jïn racha-i
Rangi rangi bati kar kar jïnsi mai-a jïn ūpa-i
Kar kar vey-key kita apna jïv tïs di vadia-i
Jo tïs bavey so-i karsi hūkam na karna ja-i
So patïsa saha patïsa-ib Nanïk rehan raja-i ||27||

Mūnda santok saram pat joli di-an ki karey bïbūt
Kinta kal ku-ari kai-a jūgat dan-da partit
Aa-i panti sagal jamati man jitey jag jit
Adeys tïsey adeys aad anil anad anahat jūg jūg eko veys ||28||

Būgat gi-an dai-a ban-daran gat gat vajey nad
Aap nat nati sab ja-ki rïd sïd avra sad
Sanjog vijog du-eh kar chalavey ley-key avey bag
Adeys tïsey adeys aad anil anad anahat jūg jūg eko veys ||29||

Eyka mai jūgat via-i tïn chey-ley parvan
Ek sansari ek bandari ek la-i diban
Jïv tïs bavey tïvey chalavey jïv hovey furman
Oh vey-key ona nadar na avey bauta e vidan
Adeys tïsey adeys aad anil anad anahat jūg jūg eko veys ||30||

50

Asan lo-e lo-e bandar
Jo kïch pai-a su eyka var
Kar kar vey-key sirjanhar
Nanïk sachey ki sachi kar
Adeys tïsey adeys aad anil anad anahat jūg jūg eko veys ||31||

Ek dū jibo lak ho-e lak hovey lak vis
Lak lak geyra aki-ey ek nam jag dis
Eyt-ra pat pavari-a chari-ey ho-eh ïkis
Sūn gala akas ki kita a-i ris
Nanïk Nadri pai-ey kūri kūrey tis ||32||

Akan jor chūpey na jor
Jor na mangan deyn na jor
Jor na jivan maran na jor
Jor na raj mal man sor
Jor na surti gi-an vichar
Jor na jūgti chūtey sansar
Jïs hat jor kar vey-key so-i
Nanïk ūtam nich na ko-I ||33||

Rati rūti tïti var
Pavan pani agni patal
Tïs vïch darti tap raki daram sal
Tïs vïch ji-a jūgat key rang
Tïn key nam aneyk anant
Karmi karmi ho-i vichar
Sacha aap sacha darbar
Tïtey sohan panch parvan
Nadri karam pavey nisan
Kach pakai o-tey pa-i
Nanïk gai-a japey ja-i ||34||

Daram kand ka ey-ho daram
Gi-an kand ka ako karam
Key-tey pavan pani vey-santar key-tey kan maheys
Key-tey barmey garat gari-ey rūp rang key veys
Keyti-a karam būmi meyr key-tey key-tey dū ūpdeys
Key-tey ïnd chand sūr key-tey key-tey mandal deys
Key-tey sïd būd nat key-tey key-tey deyvi veys
Key-tey deyv danav mūn key-tey key-tey ratan samūnd
Keyti-a kani keyti-a bani key-tey pat narïnd
Keyti-a surti seyvak key-tey Nanïk ant na ant ||35||

Gi-an kand me gi-an parchand
Tït-tey nad binod kod anand
Saram kand ki bani rūp
Tït-tey garat gari-ey baut anūp

51

Ta kia gala kati-a na ja-i
Jey ko kahey pichey pachu-tai
Tït-tey gari-ey surat mat man būd
Tït-tey gari-ey sura sïda ki sūd ||36||

Karam kand ki bani jor
Tït-tey hor na ko-i hor
Tït-tey jod mahabal sūr
Tïn mey ram rey-a barpūr
Tït-tey sito sita mahima ma-i
Ta key rūp na kat-ney ja-i
Na-o marey na tagey ja-i
Jïn key ram vasey man ma-i
Tït-tey bagat vasey key lo-a
Karey anand sacha man so-i
Sach kand vasey nirankar
Kar kar vey-key nadar nïhal
Tït-tey kand mandal varband
Jey ko katey ta ant na ant
Tït-tey lo-a lo-a akar
Jïv jïv hūkam tïvey tïv kar
vey-key vïgsey kar vichar
Nanïk katïna karara sar ||37||

Jat pahara diraj sūni-ar
Ey-ran mat veyd hati-ar
Bao kala agan tap ta-o
Banda bao amrït tït dal
Gari-ey sabd sachi taksal
Jïn kao nadar karam tïn kar
Nanïk nadri nadar nïhal ||38||

Slok
Pavan guru pani pïta mata darat mahat
Dïvas rat du-i dai dai-a key-ley sagal jagat
Changia-ia būria-ia vachey daram hadūr
Karmi apo apni key ney-rey key dūr
Jïni nam dia-ia gey masakat gal
Nanïk tey mūk ūjaley keyti chūti nal ||1||

The effects of chanting each pauri, from the teachings of Yogi Bhajan[144], are listed beneath each translation[145] *in italics.*

There is one Creator/Creation; Truth is His Name; Doer of everything, Fearless, Revengeless, Undying, Unborn, Self Illumined; This is the gift of the Guru; Recite it through Repetition True in the beginning, True through all ages, True now; Nanak says Truth shall ever be ||1||

"The Mul Mantra is a fate killer. It removes the fate and changes the destiny to prosperity"

By thinking, He cannot be reduced to thought, even by thinking over long periods of time
Though one remains silent & absorbed in God's constant love, inner silence is not obtained
The hunger of the hungry is not appeased, though they may pile up loads of worldly valuables
One may possess thousands of clever tricks, but not even one of them will go along with him
So how can you become truthful and tear away the veil of illusion?
O, Nanak, by obeying the order to the Lord's Command & Walking in the Way of His Will ||1||

"The second half of the 1st pauri will lift you from depression, insecurity, nightmares and loss"

By God's Command, bodies are created and His Command cannot be narrated
By His Command souls come into being; by His Command glory and greatness are obtained
By His Command some are high, some are low; by His written Command pain, pleasure obtained
Some, by His Command, are blessed, forgiven; others, by His Command, wander aimlessly forever
Every one is subject to His Command; no one is exempt from His Command
O, Nanak, one who understands His Command does not speak in ego ||2||

"Imparts patience and stability"

Some sing of His Might; Who has the power to sing it?
Some sing of His Gifts, and know His Sign
Some sing of His Glorious Virtues, Greatness and Beauty
Some sing of Knowledge obtained of Him, through difficult philosophical studies
Some sing that He fashions the body, and then again reduces it to dust
Some sing that He takes life away, then restores it
Some sing that He seems so very far away
Some sing that He watches over us, face to face, ever-present
There is no shortage of those who preach and teach
Millions upon millions give millions of sermons about God
The Great Giver goes on giving and the recipients grow weary of receiving
Throughout the ages the partakers partake
The Commander, by His Command, leads us to walk on the path
O, Nanak the Care-free Master blossoms forth untroubled ||3||

"Transforms insufficiency into sufficiency; turns depression into elevation; transforms low self-esteem into complete self-confidence"

True is the Lord, True His Name and the true have repeated His Name with infinite love
People beg and pray 'give to us', 'give to us' and the Great Bestower gives his Gifts
So what offering can we place before Him, where-by His court may be seen?
What words can we utter to evoke His Love?
During the Amrit Vela, the hours before dawn, chant the True Name reflect upon His Greatness
By the karma of past actions, the robe of the physical body is obtained & by Grace, Salvation found
O, Nanak, know this well: the True One Himself is All ||4||

"Blesses those trapped in feelings of poverty and lack of means. It blasts through the trap of these feelings like a thunderbolt"

He cannot be established nor created by anyone
He Himself is Immaculate and Pure

Those who serve Him are honored
O, Nanak sing of the Lord, the Treasure of Excellence
Sing and listen, and let your mind be filled with love
Your pain shall be sent far away and peace shall come to your home
The Guru's Word is the Sacred Sound Current of the Nad, Wisdom of the Vedas & all-pervading
The Guru is Shiva, the Guru is Vishnu, the Guru is Brahma; the Guru is Parvati and Lakshmi
Even knowing God, I cannot describe Him; He cannot be described by words
The Guru has given me this one understanding:
There is only the One, the Giver of all souls; may I never forget him! ||5||

"The 5th pauri must be recited when you feel a sense of failure within yourself; When you feel that you are not up to the job, this pauri will grant you success"

If I am pleasing to Him, that is my pilgrimage bath; without pleasing Him, what good are rituals?
I gaze upon the created beings; without the karma of good actions, what do they receive?
Within the mind are gems, jewels and rubies, if you listen to the Guru's teachings, even once
The Guru has given me this one understanding:
There is only the One. The Giver of all souls; may I never forget Him! ||6||

"Dispels limitation; Recite it when you feel limited, cornered, trapped or coerced"

Even if you could live throughout the four ages, or grow ten times more
And even if you were known throughout the nine continents and followed by all
With a good name and reputation, with praise and fame throughout the world
Still, if the Lord does not bless you with His Glance of Grace, then who cares?
You would be but a vermin amongst worms and even sinners would hold you in contempt
O, Nanak God grants virtue to the un-virtuous and bestows piety upon the pious
I can think of no such one who can even imagine anyone who can bestow virtue upon Him ||7||

"When you suffer from greed, madness for power, overbearing expansion and the need to control; when you become trapped in your territoriality, this pauri will heal you"

By listening, the mere mortal becomes the spiritual teacher, the heroic yogi, the great master
By listening, the earth and the akashic ether is revealed
By listening, the knowledge of the oceans, lands of the world & nether regions of the underworld
By listening, death cannot even touch you
By listening, sorrow and sin find their destruction ||8||

"Gives the power to be a perfect sage"

By listening, the knowing of Shiva, Brahma & Indra are obtained
By listening, find that the evil-tongued even speak praises of his name
By listening, one attains the understanding of the way of Yoga and the secrets of the body
By listening, knowledge of the Shastras, Simritees and Vedas is acquired
O, Nanak ever blissful are the devotees
By listening, disease and wickedness are erased ||9||

"Gives expansion"

By listening, truth, contentment and Divine Knowledge are obtained
By listening, the fruits of bathing at the 68 pilgrimage sites are attained

By listening, reading and reciting one gains honor
By listening, one intuitively grasps the essence of meditation
O, Nanak ever blissful are the devotees
By listening, disease and wickedness are erased ||10||

"Grants Grace"

By listening, one dives deep into the ocean of virtues
By listening, the mortal is rendered a scholar, spiritual guide and emperor
By listening, the blind find the way
By listening, the unattainable comes within your reach
O, Nanak ever blissful are the devotees
By listening, disease and wickedness are erased ||11||

"Gives virtuousness"

The state of the faithful cannot be described
One who tries to describe it shall regret the attempt
No paper, no pen, no scribe
Can record the state of the faithful
Such is the Name of the Immaculate Lord
Only one who has faith comes to know such a state of mind ||12||

"When you feel small, this pauri gives you solidarity of self, self-impressiveness and self-respect"

The faithful have intuitive awareness and understanding
The faithful attain the knowledge of the spheres
The faithful shall never be struck across the face
The faithful do not have to answer to the Messenger of Death
Such is the Name of the Immaculate Lord
Only one who has faith comes to know such a state of mind ||13||

"Gives you the occult knowledge of infinity; It brings deep intuition"

The faithful's path shall never be obstructed
The faithful depart with honor and renown
The faithful do not follow hollow religious rituals
The faithful has an alliance with righteousness
Such is the Name of the Immaculate Lord
Only one who has faith comes to know such a state of mind ||14||

"When you cannot find your path in life, when you cannot see the direction to your destiny, and when you cannot achieve fulfillment, this pauri will show you the way"

The faithful finds the door of liberation
The faithful redeem and reform their kin
The faithful are saved and save the students of the Guru
The faithful do not wander around begging
Such is the Name of the Immaculate Lord
Only one who has faith comes to know such a state of mind ||15||

The chosen ones are self-elected, accepted and approved
The chosen ones are honored in the Court of the Lord
The chosen look beautiful in the courts of kings
The chosen meditate single-mindedly on the Guru
No matter how much someone tries to explain and describe it
There can be no enumeration of the Creator's doing
Dharma is the mythical bull, the offspring of compassion
This holds the earth in order
How great is the load that the bull carries?
The one who understands this becomes True
There are many worlds beyond this earth
What power is there which supports their weight from beneath?
The names and colors of the many beings and species
Were all inscribed by the ever-flowing pen of God
Who holds the knowledge to write this account?
Imagine how voluminous the scroll would be
What power and fascinating beauty!
How great Thy Gift! Who can even assess it?
You created the vast expanse of the Universe with One Word
Whereby innumerable rivers began to flow
What power have I to describe Your Creative Potency?
I cannot even be a sacrifice unto Thee
Whatever pleases You is what is good
Thou art ever safe and sound, O Formless One ||16||

"Gives knowledge of the structure of the universe"

Countless meditation, countless love
Countless worship services, countless disciplines
Countless scriptures and ritual recitation of the Vedas
Countless yogis, whose minds detach from the world
Countless devotees contemplate Your Wisdom and Virtues
Countless are the holy, countless the givers
Countless warriors who eat steel with their mouths and bear the brunt on their faces
Countless are the silent sages who vibrate the String of Gods Love
I cannot even be a sacrifice unto Thee
Whatever pleases You is what is good
Thou art ever safe and sound, O Formless One ||17||

"Brings freedom and resurrection"

Countless fools blinded by ignorance
Countless thieves and embezzlers
Countless impose their will by force
Countless who cut throats and murder
Countless sinners who continue to sin
Countless liars who wander in falsehood
Countless wretches who eat filth as their ration
Countless slanderers who carry the weight of their sins on their heads
Nanak describes the state of the lowly

I cannot even be a sacrifice unto Thee
Whatever pleases You is what is good
Thou art ever safe and sound, O Formless One ||18||

"Fights madness, deep feelings of inferiority and self-destructive behavior"

Countless Names, countless places
Countless are the inaccessible realms
Even to call them countless is to carry the weight on your head
From the Word comes the Nam, from the Word comes Your Praise
From the Word comes spiritual wisdom, singing the Songs of Your Glory
From the Word come the written and spoken hymns
From the Word comes destiny inscribed on one's forehead
But the One who wrote this destiny bears no words on His Forehead
As He ordains, so do we receive
The Universe is the manifestation of Thy Name
Without Thy Name, there is no place at all
What power have I to describe Your Creative Potency?
I cannot even be a sacrifice unto Thee
Whatever pleases You is what is good
Thou art ever safe and sound, O Formless One ||19||

"Brings universal knowledge, inspiration and revelation"

When the hands, feet and body are dirty
Water can wash away the dirt
When the garments are soiled with urine
Soap can wash them clean
When the mind is stained and polluted with sin
It can only be cleansed by the Love of God's Name
A human does not become virtuous or vicious by mere words of mouth
Repeated actions are engraved on the soul
You shall reap what it is you have sowed
O Nanak, by God's Command, men come and go (in reincarnation) ||20||

"When the monsters are nipping at your heels, this pauri wipes away all your sins"

Pilgrimage, disciplines, compassion and charity
These by themselves, bring but a sesame (an iota) of merit
By listening to God's Name with love and humility
One obtains the salvation of bathing at the shrine deep within the self
All Virtues are Yours, Lord; I have not myself
Without virtues, there is no form of devotional worship
I am obedient to the Lord of the World, to His Word, to Brahma the Creator
He is Beautiful, True and rapture ever abides within His Mind
What was the time, the moment, what lunar day, what week day?
And what was the season and month that the Universe was created?
The Pandits, religious scholars, cannot find that time, even though it is written in the Puranas
Nor do the Qazis, who scribe the Koran, know this time
Neither the Yogis nor anyone else, know the lunar day, week day, season or month
Only the Creator who creates the world knows
How to express, how to praise, how to describe, how to know Thee

O, Nanak many speak of Him, each wiser than the next
Great is the Master, Great His Name and whatever happens is according to his will
O, Nanak one who claims to know all shall not be adorned upon arrival in the afterworld ||21||

"Will maintain your status, grace and position"

There are nether worlds and hundreds of thousands of heavenly worlds above
The Vedas say that you can search and search for them all until you grow weary
The Semitic scriptures say that there are 18,000 worlds, but there is only one Limitless Lord
If one tried to write an account of this, the end of man would precede the end of the account
O, Nanak call Him Great! Only He Himself knows Himself ||22||

"Brings victory in legal battles; it gives you the strategy"

The praisers praise the Lord but they do not attain His understanding
They understand His extent only as well as rivers and streams know the extent of the ocean
Even kings and emperors with mountains of property and oceans of wealth
Equal not to an ant who does not forget the True Lord ||23||

"Dispels darkness and elevates the self"

Limitless are His Praises to those who speak them
Limitless are His Actions and limitless His Gifts
Limitless His Vision, limitless His Hearing
His Limits cannot be described; what is His Motivation?
The limits of the created universe cannot be perceived
The limit of His will here and beyond is unknown
Many struggle to know His limits
But this limit none can know
The more we attempt to describe, the more obscure it becomes
Great is the Master, High is His Heavenly Throne
Highest of the high, above all is His Name
Only one as Great and as High as God
Can know the Exalted State of the Lofty Being
How Great He is, only He Himself knows
O, Nanak by His Grace, Blessings are bestowed ||24||

"Breaks through all limitations with the force of a thunderbolt, so powerfully that it affects generations; it has the power to kill misfortune"

So abundant are His Blessings that there can be no account of them
The Great Giver has no idea of avarice
Many great warriors beg at the Door of the Infinite Lord
Many contemplate upon Him, that they cannot be counted
Many waste away engaged in corruption
Many take and take but deny receiving
Many foolish consumers continue consuming
Many endure distress, hunger and constant abuse
Even these are Thy Gifts, Great Giver
Liberation from bondage comes only from God's Will
No other has a say in this
If some fool should presume to say that he does

They shall learn and feel the effects of their folly
The Lord Himself knows, Himself gives
Very few are those who acknowledge this
One who is blessed to sing the Praises of the Lord
O, Nanak is the king of kings ||25||

"When you recite this pauri, all your needs become pre-fulfilled; Prosperity, virtue, estate and wealth are yours without asking"

Priceless are Thine Virtues, priceless Thine Dealings
Priceless are Thine Dealers, priceless Thine Treasures
Priceless are those who come to You and priceless are those who buy from You
Priceless is Thy Affection, priceless is absorption into Thee
Priceless is Thy Divine Law of Dharma, priceless is Thy Court of Justice
Priceless are Thine Scales, priceless Thine Weights
Priceless Thine Gifts, priceless Thy Mark of approval
Priceless Thy Mercy, priceless Thy Command
Priceless beyond value, beyond expression!
Speak continually of God and remain absorbed in His Love
The reciters of the Vedas and Puranas proclaim
Scholars speak and lecture upon God's Name
Brahmas and Indras speak God's Name
The Gopis and Krishna speak
Shiva and the Siddhas speak
All the Buddhas created by God speak
The demons speak and the demi-gods speak
The heavenly beings, silent sages and servants speak of God
Many speak and attempt to describe Him
Many have spoken of Him repeatedly and have then arisen and departed
If God were to create as many as there already are
Even then, they could not describe Him
The Lord becomes as Great as He pleases
O, Nanak only the True Lord knows
If anyone says they can describe God
He shall be known as the greatest fool of all fools! ||26||

"Transforms nothing into everything; In your business it vanishes losses, misfortunes and miseries"

Where is the Gate and where is the Dwelling in which You sit and take care of all?
The Sacred Sound Current vibrates there & countless musicians play on various instruments there
So many Ragas, so many musicians singing there
The wind, water and fire sing and the Righteous Judge of Dharma sings at Your Door
Angels of consciousness (Chitra & Gupat) record actions and the Righteous Judge of Dharma sing
Shiva, Brahma and the Goddess of Beauty, ever adorned, sing
Indra, seated upon His Throne, sings with the deities at Thy Gate
In Samadhi, the Siddhas sing; In contemplation, the Saddhus sing
The celibates, the content and the accepting sing
The Pandits, those who recited the Vedas, together with the 7 supreme sages, sing
The Mohinis, enchanting beauties who entice hearts in paradise and in the subconscious, sing
The 14 celestial jewels and the 68 holy places of pilgrimage sing
The brave and mighty warriors sing; the 4 sources of creation sing
The continents, planets and solar systems, created and arranged by Your Hand, sing

They alone sing who please Your Will; Your devotees are imbued with the Nectar of Your Name
So many others sing, they do not come to mind; O, Nanak, how can I consider them all?
That and that Lord is ever True, His is True, and True is His Name
He is & shall always be; He shall not depart even when this Universe, which He created, departs
He created the world, with its various colors, species of beings and the variety of Maya (illusions)
Having created the Creation, He watches over it Himself, by His Greatness
He does whatever he pleases; no order can be issued to Him
He is the King, The King of kings; Nanak remains subject to His Will ||27||

"When you are stuck and cannot see the window of opportunity before you; this pauri shows you the way; It removes obstacles so you can leap over hurdles"

Let contentment be your ear-rings, humility your begging bowl, meditation ashes upon your body
Thought of death your patched coat, purity of the virgin your way & The Lord your walking stick
Make brotherhood the highest order of yoga; Deem the conquer of the self as conquering the world
I bow to Him, I humbly bow
The Primal One is without beginning, the unstruck sound, whose form is one through all ages ||28||

"The strongest permutation and combination of words in the world; It unites God"

Make Divine Knowledge your food, compassion your steward; the Nad beats in every heart
He Himself is the Supreme; wealth, miracles and spiritual powers are but beads on a string
Union and separation come by His Will; We come to receive what is written in our destiny
I bow to Him, I humbly bow
The Primal One is without beginning, the unstruck sound, whose form is one through all ages ||29||

"A shield of protection from enemies; It vaporizes animosity towards you"

The One Divine Mother conceived and gave birth to the 3 deities
One, Creator of the World (Brahma); One, the Sustainer (Vishnu): One, the Destroyer (Shiva)
He makes things happen according to the Pleasure of His Will
He watches over all but none see him; this is the greatest wonder!
I bow to Him, I humbly bow
The Primal One is without beginning, the unstruck sound, whose form is one through all ages ||30||

"Places you upon the throne of divinity; It makes you into a sage and a saint"

The Lord's Seat and Storehouses are in all the worlds
Whatever was put in them was put there once and for all
Having created the creation, the Lord is watching over it
O, Nanak True is the work of the True Lord
I bow to Him, I humbly bow
The Primal One is without beginning, the unstruck sound, whose form is one through all ages ||31||

"Pulls all virtues from the heavens"

If I had 100,000 tongues, and those were then multiplied 20 times more, with each tongue
I would repeat 100's of 1,000's of times the Name of the One Lord of the Universe
Along this path to our Husband Lord, we ascend the steps of the ladder & come to merge with Him
Hearing of the etheric realm, even vermin long to come back home
O, Nanak God is obtained by His Grace; false are the boastings of the false ||32||

"Pays your debts and completes your karma"

I have no power to speak, no power to remain silent
I have no power to beg, no power to give
I have no power to live, no power to die
I have no power to acquire wealth which stirs up commotion in the mind
I have no power to gain understanding of Divine Knowledge
I have no power to find the way to escape from the world
God alone, has the Power in His Hands as He excercises and beholds it
O Nanak, by one's own strength, none can be high or low ||33||

"Destroys your ego and brings forth your divinity; It removes negativity, neutralizes your destructive nature and prevents harm to others by your hand"

God created nights, days, weeks and seasons
Wind, water, fire and the nether regions
In the midst of these, He established the earth as a home for Dharma, the way of life
There He placed beings of various types and colors
Various and endless are their names
By their deeds and actions they shall be judged
God Himself is True and True His Court
There, in perfect grace and ease, sit the self-elect, the self-realized Saints
They receive the Mark of Grace of the Merciful Master
The ripe and unripe, the good and the bad, shall be judged
O, Nanak upon arrival Home, you will see this ||34||

"Brings stability"

The aforementioned is moral duty in the realm of Dharma (righteous living)
Now, I speak in the realm of Spiritual Knowledge
So many winds, waters and fires; so many Krishnas and Shivas
So many Brahmas fashioning forms and beauties adorned and dressed in many colors
So many worlds and lands for resolving karmas; so very many lessons to be learned
So many Indras, moons and suns; so many worlds and lands
So many Siddhas, Buddhas & Yogic Masters; so very many forms of Goddesses
So many deities, demons and silent sages; so very many oceans of jewels
So many ways of living, so many languages, so many dynasties of kings
So many people of Divine Knowledge, so many servants of God; O, Nanak He has no limit ||35||

"Gives you the capacity to do your duty and fulfill your responsibility"

In the realm of knowledge, Spiritual Wisdom reigns supreme
The Nad vibrates amidst the sounds and the sights of bliss
Beauty is the language in the realm of spirit
Forms of an incomparable beauty are fashioned there
The proceedings of that place cannot be described
One who attempts to speak of these shall regret the endeavor
The inner consciousness, intellect and understanding of the mind are molded there
There, the consciousness of the pious & the Siddhas, beings performing miracles, are shaped ||36||

"Brings divine realization; it grants complete understanding of the Heavens and the Earth"

In the realm of Karma, the word is Power
No one else dwells there
Except for the warriors of great power and heroes
They are totally fulfilled, imbued with the Lord's Esssence
The Sitas are there, cool and calm in their majestic glory
Their beauty cannot be described
Neither death nor deception comes to those
Within whose minds the Lord abides
The saints of many worlds dwell there
They celebrate; their minds are imbued with the True Lord
In the realm of Truth the Formless Lord abides
Having created the creation, He watches over it and bestows happiness by His Glance of Grace
In that realm there are planets, solar systems and galaxies
If one attempts to describe them, they should know that these have no limits or bounds
There are universes upon universes of His Creation
As He commands, so they exist
The Lord watches over all, and contemplating the creation, He rejoices
O, Nanak to describe this is as hard as iron! ||37||

"Cuts the karma; it eliminates the impact of all bad karmas"

Let self-control be your furnace and patience the goldsmith
Let understanding be the anvil and Spiritual Wisdom the tool
Let the fear of God be the bellows to fan the flames of tapas, the body's inner heat
Let the Love of the Lord be your crucible whereby you make molten the Necar of the Name
Thus, in the minting process, the True Coin of the Shabad, the Word of God
Such is the karma of those upon whom God casts His Gracious Glance
O, Nanak the Merciful Lord, by His Grace, uplifts and exalts them ||38||

"Gives you the power to rewrite your own destiny"

Final Sermon (Slok)
Air is the Guru, water the Father, earth the Great Mother
Day and night are the two nurses, in whose lap all the world is at play
The record of good deeds and bad deeds is read out in the presence of the Lord of Dharma
According to their own actions, some are drawn closer and some are driven further away
Those who have meditated on the Nam & departed having worked by the sweat of their brows
O, Nanak their faces are radiant in the Lord's Court & many shall be liberated along with them ||1||

"Brings self-satisfaction, elevation, acknowledgment and respect"

SHABD HAZAREY

Shabd Hazarey was initially composed in a series of 3 letters, which represent the first 3 stanzas, from *Arjan* (who later became the Fifth Guru) to his Beloved Guru and Father, *Guru Ram Das*. The 3 letters were written from a place of profound love and devotion while the two were separated (*Arjan* was sent by his father to attend to a family wedding on his behalf). Upon reunion, *Guru Ram Das* told his son to create a fourth stanza, thus completing the poem.[146] The opening lines of Shabd Hazarey (known as *Mere Man Lochey*) were taught by Yogi Bhajan as the *Meditation to Heal the Wounds of Love*[147].

Here is what he once spoke about this *bani*:

Those words are very powerful to connect the conscious, unconscious, and subconscious and bring the formality of love to the extent that Guru Ram Das gave Guru Arjun Dev the Guruship. He was Arjanmal but he became Guru Arjun. People sing *mere man lochey*; you can take a recording of it and play with it. It does work and it has no failing record. When anybody is abandoned by love or lover, or there's someone he wants to meet, unite and put together, if you read that *Shabd Hazarey* everyday and sing it, playing it eleven times a day as a sadhana, a personal sadhana, it brings you victory.[148]

Maj Mehla Panjva (5) Cha-ūpdey Ghar Pehila (1)

Mere Man Lochey Gur Darshan Ta-i
Bïlap Karey Chatrik Ki Nia-i
Trika Na Utarey Sant Na Avey
Bïn Darshan Sant Pi-arey Jio
Ho Goli Jio Gol Gūma-i
Gur Darshan Sant Pi-arey Jio ||1|| Rahao

Teyra Mūk Suhava Ji-o Sahaj Dūn Bani
Chir Ho-a Deykey Sarïng Pani
Dan So Deys Jaha Tu Vasi-a
Meyrey Sajan Mit Murarey Jio
Ho Goli Ho Gol Guma-i
Gur Sajan Mit Murarey Jio ||2|| Rahao

Ik Gari Na Milatey Ta Kalijūg Hota
Hūn Kad Mili-ai Prai-a Tūd Bagavanta
Mo-eh Ren Na Vihavey Nid Na Avey
Bïn Deykey Gur Darbarey Jio
Ho Goli Jio Gol Gūma-i
Tïs Sachey Gur Darbarey Jio ||3|| Rahao

Bag Ho-a Gur Sant Mïlai-a
Prab Abinasi Gar Meh Pai-a
Seyv Kari Pal Chasa Na Vichura
Jan Nanïk Das Tūmarey Jio ||4||
Ho Goli Jio Gol Gūma-i

63

Jan Nanïk Das Tūmarey Jio ||1||8||

Danasri Mehla Pehila (1)
Ghar Pehila (1) Cha-ūpdey

Ek Ong Kar
Sat Nam
Karta Purk
Nirbhao Nir-ver
Akal Mūrït
Ajūni Saibang
Gūr Prasad

Jio Darat Hey Apna Key
Sio Kari Pūkar
Dūk Vïsaran Seyvia
Sada Sada Datar ||1||
Sahïb Meyra Nit Nava
Sada Sada Datar ||1||

Rahao

Andïn Sahïb Seyvi-ey
Ant Shada-ey So-ey
Sūn Sūn Meyri Kamni
Par Utara Ho-ey ||2||
Dai-al Tey-rey Nam Tara
Sad Kurbaney Jao ||1||

Rahao

Sarbang Sacha Eyk Hey
Dūja Nahi Ko-ey
Taki Seyva So Karey Ja
Kao Nadr Karey ||3||
Tūd Baj Piarey Keyv Raha
Sa Vadia-i De Jït Nam
Tey-Rey Lag Raha
Dūja Nahi Ko-ey Jïs
Agey Pi-aray Ja-ey Kaha ||1||

Rahao

Seyvi Sahïb Apna
Avar Na Jacha-o Ko-ey
Nanïk Taka Das He
Bïnd-bïnd Chūk-chūk Ho-ey ||4||
Sahïb Tey-rey Nam Vït-hau
Bïnd Bïnd Chūk Chūk Ho-ey ||1||

Rahao ||4||1||

Tilang Mehla Pehila Ghar Tija (3)

Ek Ong Kar Satigur Prasad
Ehu Tan Mai-a Pahi-a
Pi-arey Litra Lab Ranga-ey
Mey-rey Kant Na-bavey Chol-ra
Piarey Kio Dan Sey-jey Ja-e ||1||
Hau Kurbaney Jao
Mirvana Hau Kurbaney Jao
Hau Kurbaney Jao Tina Key
Lae Jo Teyra Nao
Len Jo Teyra Nao
Tina Key Hau Sad Kurbaney Jao ||1||

Rahao

Kai-a Rangan Jey Ti-ey
Pi-arey Pai-ey Nao Majit
Rangan Vala Jey Rangey
Sahib Eysa Rang Na Dit ||2||
Jin Key Choley Rat-rey
Pi-arey Kant Tina Key Pas
Dur Tina Ki Jey Miley Ji
Kaho Nanik Ki Ardas ||3||
Apey Sajey Apey Rangey
Apey Nadr Kare-e
Nanik Kamin Kante Bavey
Apey Hi Rave-e ||4||1||3||

Tilang Mehla Pehila (1)

E-an Re-ey Manra
Ka-ey Karey-he
Aap Nar-hey Gar Har
Rango Ki Na Mane-he
Saho Ney-rey Dan Kamli-ey
Bahar Kia Dundey-he
Bhai Kia De Sala-ia
Neyni Bav Ka Kar Sigaro
Ta Sohagan Jani-ey
Lagi Ja Saho Darey Pi-aro ||1||

E-ani Bali Kia Karey
Ja Dan Kant Na Bavey
Karn Pala Karey Bau
Tey-rey Sa Dan Mahal Na Pavey
Vin Karma Kich Pai-ey Nahi
Jey Bau-teyra Davey
Lab Lob Ahang-kar Ki
Mati Mai-a Mahi Samani

Eni Bati Sao Pai-ey
Nahi Bhey Kamïn I-ani ||2||

Ja-ey Pūchau Sohag-ni
Va-e Kïni Bati Saho Pai-ey
Jo Kich Karey So Bala Kar
Mani-ey Hïkmat Hūkam Chūkai-ey
Ja Key Parem Padart Pai-ey
To Charni Chït Lai-ey
Saho Kahey So Kijey Tan Mano
Dijey Eysa Parmal Lai-ey
Eyv Kahey Sohag-ni Bhey-ney
Ini Bati Saho Pai-ey ||3||

Aap Gavai-ey Ta Saho
Pai-ey A-or Keysi Chatura-i
Saho Nadr Kar Dey-key Sodïn
Ley-key Kamïn Nao Nïd Pa-e
Apney Kant Pi-ari Sa
Sohagïn Nanïk Sa Sabrha-i
Ey-sey Rang Rati Sahej Ki
Mati Eynïs Ba-ey Samani
Sūndr Sa-ey Sarūp Bïch-kan
Kai-ey Sasi-ani ||4||2||4||

Sūh-i Mehla Pehila (1)

Kaun Taraji Kavan Tula
Teyra Kavan Sarf Būlava
Kaun Guru Key Pe Diki-a
Leyva Key-pehi Mūl Karava ||1||
Mey-rey Lal Jio Teyra Ant-na Jana
Tūn Jal-tal Mey-hi-al Baripur
Lina Tūn Apey Sarab Samana ||1||

Rahao

Man Taraji Chït Tula
Teyri Seyv Saraf Kamava
Gat-hi Bitar So Saho
Toli-in Bïd Chït Rahava ||2||
Apey Kanda Tol Taraji
Apey Tolïn-hara
Apey Dey-kae Apey Būjey
Apey Hey Vanjara ||3||
Andula Nich Jat Pardeysi
Kïn Avey Tïl Javey
Taki Sangat Nanïk Rada
Kio Kar Mūra Pavey ||4||2||9||

Ek Ong Kar
Sat Nam
Karta Purk
Nirbhao Nir-ver
Akal Mūrït
Ajūni Saibang
Gūr Prasad

Rag Bïlaval Mehla Pehila (1)
Cha-ūpdey Gar Pehila (1)

Tu Sūltan Kaha Hao
Mia Teyri Kavan Vada-i
Jo Tu-de So Kaha Su-ami
Mey Murk Kehan-na Jai ||1||
Tey-rey Gūn Gava De Būja-i
Je-sey Sach Me Rahao Raja-i ||1||

Rahao

Jo Kich Hoa Sab Kich
Tūj-tey Tey-rey Sab Asna-i
Teyra Ant Na Jana Mey-rey
Sahïb Mey Anduley Kia Chatura-i ||2||
Kia Hao Kati Katey Kat
Deyka Mey Akat-na Katna Jai
Jo Tūd Bhavey So-i Aka
Tïl Teyri Vadi-ai ||3||
Eytey Kūkar Hao Beygana
Ba-uka Istan Tai
Bagat-hïn Nanïk Je Ho-ega
Ta Kasmey Nao Na Jai ||4||1||

Bïlaval Mehla Pehila (1)

Man Mandr Tan Veys Kalandr
Gat Hi Tirat Nava
Eyk Sabd Mey-rey Pran Bast
Hey Bahur Janam Na-ava ||1||
Man Beydi-a Dai-al
Seyti Meyri Mai
Kaun Janey Pir Para-i
Ham Na-i Chïnt Para-i ||1||

Rahao

Agam Agochar Alak Apara
Chïnta Karau Hamari
Jal Tal Mahi-el Baripur Lina
Ghat Ghat Jot Tūm Hari ||2||

Sïk Mat Sab Būd Tūm-hari
Mandir Chava Tey-rey
Tūj Bïn Avar-na Jana Mey-rey
Sai-ba Gūn Gava Nït Tey-rey ||3||
Jia Jant Sab Saran Tūm-hari
Sarab Chïnt Tūd Pasey
Jo Tūd Bavey So-i Changa
Ek Nanïk Ki Arda-sey ||4||2||

Maj, Fifth Mehl, Four Lines per Hymn, First House of Rag
(These denote which Rag, or musical melodic structure, is to be applied to the following stanza & from which Guru this hymn comes.)

My mind longs for the Guru's Darshan (the sight of the Guru). It cries out like the thirsty song bird for the nectar of your name. My thirst is not quenched, and I can not find peace until I receive the Darshan of the beloved saint. ||1||Pause||
(The purpose of each Rahao, or Pause, is to allow a moment to contemplate what has just been read)

I give myself, and my soul for your Darshan, my beloved Guru! Your face is so beautiful, and the sound of your words (shabd) is so filled with inner wisdom. It has been too long since this rain bird has had even a glimpse of water. Blessed is the land where you live, my friend and loved one, my Divine Teacher. ||2||Pause||

I give myself, and my soul, to my beloved, my Divine Guru. An instant away from you, brings darkness. When will I meet You, my beloved Wahe Guru? I can't endure this night, sleep eludes me too until I see your home, my beloved Guru! ||3||Pause||

I give myself, and my soul to your true home, my beloved Guru! By good fortune, I met my Saint Guru and I have found that the immortal creator is within the home of my own self and so I will always serve you and never be separated from you even for an instant. Guru Nanak says: I'm your slave, my beloved Lord. ||4||
I give myself and my soul. Servant Nanak lives to serve you. ||1||8||
Danasri, from the First Guru, First House of Rag, Four Lines per Hymn

One Creator, Creation; Truth is His Name. Doer of everything. Fearless, Revengeless, Undying, Unborn, Self Illumined. It is by Guru's Grace. My soul is afraid; to whom should I complain? I serve Him, who makes me forget my pains; He is the Giver, forever and ever. ||1||
My Lord and Master is forever new; He is the Giver, forever and ever. ||1||Pause||

Night and day, I serve my Lord and Master; He shall save me in the end. Hearing and listening, O my dear sister, I have crossed over. ||2||

O Merciful Lord, Your Name carries me across. I am forever a sacrifice to You. ||1||Pause||
In all the world, there is only the One True Lord; there is no other at all. He alone serves the Lord, upon whom the Lord casts His Glance of Grace. ||3||

Without You, O Beloved, how could I even live? Bless me with such greatness, that I may remain attached to Your Name. There is no other, O Beloved, to whom I can go and speak. ||1||Pause||
I serve my Lord and Master; I ask for no other. Nanak is His slave; moment by moment, bit by bit, he is a sacrifice to Him. ||4||

O Lord Master, I am a sacrifice to Your Name, moment by moment, bit by bit. ||1||Pause||4||1||

Tilang, from the First Guru, Third House of Rag

One Universal Creator God; By The Grace Of The True Guru

This body fabric is conditioned by Maya, O Beloved; this cloth is dyed in greed. My Husband Lord is not pleased by these clothes, O Beloved; how can the soul-bride go to His bed? ||1||
I am a sacrifice, O Dear Merciful Lord; I am a sacrifice to You. I am a sacrifice to those who take to Your Name. Unto those who take to Your Name, I am forever a sacrifice. ||1||Pause||

If the body becomes the dyer's vat, O Beloved, and the Name is placed within it as the dye, and if the Dyer who dyes this cloth is the Lord Master - O, such a color has never been seen before! ||2||

Those whose shawls are so dyed, O Beloved, their Husband Lord is always with them. Bless me with the dust of those humble beings, O Dear Lord. Says Nanak, this is my prayer. ||3||

He Himself creates, and He Himself imbues us. He Himself bestows His Glance of Grace. O Nanak, if the soul-bride becomes pleasing to her Husband Lord, He Himself enjoys her. ||4||1||3||

Tilang, from the First Guru

O foolish and ignorant soul-bride, why are you so proud? Within the home of your own self, why do you not enjoy the Love of your Lord? Your Husband Lord is so very near, O foolish bride; why do you search for Him outside? Apply the Fear of God as the mascara to adorn your eyes, and make the Love of the Lord your ornament. Then, you shall be known as a devoted and committed soul-bride, when you enshrine love for your Husband Lord. ||1||

What can the silly young bride do, if she is not pleasing to her Husband Lord? She may plead and implore so many times, but still, such a bride shall not obtain the Mansion of the Lord's Presence. Without the karma of good deeds, nothing is obtained, although she may run around frantically. She is intoxicated with greed, pride and egotism, and engrossed in Maya. She cannot obtain her Husband Lord in these ways; the young bride is so foolish! ||2||

Go and ask the happy, pure soul-brides, how did they obtain their Husband Lord? Whatever the Lord does, accept that as good; do away with your own cleverness and self-will. By His Love, true wealth is obtained; link your consciousness to His lotus feet. As your Husband Lord directs, so you must act; surrender your body and mind to Him, and apply this perfume to yourself. So speaks the happy soul-bride, O sister; in this way, the Husband Lord is obtained. ||3||

Give up your selfhood, and so obtain your Husband Lord; what other clever tricks are of any use? When the Husband Lord looks upon the soul-bride with His Gracious Glance, that day is historic - the bride obtains the nine treasures. She who is loved by her Husband Lord, is the true soul-bride; O Nanak, she is the queen of all. Thus she is imbued with His Love, intoxicated with delight; day and night, she is absorbed in His Love. She is beautiful, glorious and brilliant; she is known as truly wise. ||4||2||4||

Suhi, from the First Guru

What scale, what weights, and what assayer shall I call for You, Lord? From what guru should I receive instruction? By whom should I have Your value appraised? ||1||

O my Dear Beloved Lord, Your limits are not known. You pervade the water, the land, and the sky; You Yourself are All-pervading. ||1||Pause||

Mind is the scale, consciousness the weights, and the performance of Your service is the appraiser. Deep within my heart, I weigh my Husband Lord; in this way I focus my consciousness. ||2||

You Yourself are the balance, the weights and the scale; You Yourself are the weigher. You Yourself see, and You Yourself understand; You Yourself are the trader. ||3||

The blind, low class, wandering soul comes for a moment, and departs in an instant. In its company, Nanak dwells; how can the fool attain the Lord? ||4||2||9||

One Universal Creator God. Truth Is The Name. Creative Being Personified. No Fear. No Hatred. Image Of The Undying. Beyond Birth. Self-Existent. By Guru's Grace.

Bilaval, from the First Guru, Cha-ūpdey, First House

You are the Emperor, I call You a Chief - how does this add to Your greatness? As You permit me, I praise You, O Lord Master; I am ignorant, and I cannot chant Your Praises. ||1||
Please bless me with such understanding, that I may sing Your Glorious Praises. May I dwell in Truth, according to Your Will. ||1||Pause||

Whatever has happened has all come from You. You are All-Knowing. Your limits cannot be known, O my Lord and Master; I am blind - what wisdom do I have? ||2||

What should I say? While talking, I talk of seeing, but I cannot describe the indescribable. As it pleases Your Will, I speak; it is just the tiniest bit of Your greatness. ||3||

Among so many dogs, I am an outcast; I bark for my body's belly. Without devotional worship, O Nanak, even so, still, my Master's Name does not leave me. ||4||1||

Bilaval, from the First Guru

My mind is the temple, and my body is the simple cloth of the humble seeker; deep within my heart, I bathe at the sacred shrine. The One Word of the Shabd abides within my mind; I shall not come to be born again. ||1||

My mind is pierced through by the Merciful Lord, O my mother! Who can know the pain of another? I think of none other than the Lord. ||1||Pause||

O Lord, inaccessible, unfathomable, invisible and infinite: please, take care of me! In the water, on the land and in sky, You are totally pervading. Your Light is in each and every heart. ||2||

All teachings, instructions and understandings are Yours; the mansions and sanctuaries are Yours as well. Without You, I know no other, O my Lord and Master; I continually sing Your Glorious Praises. ||3||

All beings and creatures seek the Protection of Your Sanctuary; all thought of their care rests with You. That which pleases Your Will is good; this alone is Nanak's prayer. ||4||2||[149]

JAP SAHIB

Jap Sahib is a rythmic prayer that was composed by Guru Gobind Singh, the Tenth Sikh Guru. This Hymn describes in detail God as The Divine Essence of all, the One to Whom we must bow. Simultaneously, God is poetically represented by hundreds of examples of unique, manifest forms from which all mental and perceiveable impressions during human life arise. *Jap Sahib* is chanted by devoted Sikhs in the early morning hours. It is the first bani, or hymn of *Dasam Granth* (Book of the Tenth Emperor), which is a collection of scriptures from Guru Gobind Singh. Contained within *Jap Sahib* (often written as *Jaap Sahib*), are the beloved Kundalini Yoga mantras *Chatr Chakr Varti* (stanza ||199|| - *pg. 10*) & *Ajai Alai* (stanzas ||189|| - ||196|| - *pg. 5*). **Jap** (or *japa*) is a form of meditation in which one repeats the name of God.

If you learn to pronounce Jap Sahib, God will give you power to speak and listen well. A person who does not know hoe to listen can never improve himself. And a person who cannot learn to speak cannot improve anything. Power is the word, how you receive it and how you deliver it. Power is the word.[150]

Ek Ong Kar Satïgur Prasad Jap
Sïri Mukvak Pat-Sahey
Chapai Chand Tav Prasad
Chakra Chïhn Ar Baran Jat
Ar Pat Nehïn Je
Rūp Rang Ar Reyk Beyk
Ku-ke-na Sakat Ke
Achal Mūrat Anabo Prakash
Amitoj Kahe-jey
Kot Indr Indran
Sahu Sahan Gane-jey
Tribavan Mahïp Sur Nar Asur
Net Net Ban Tren Kahet
Tav Sarab Nam Kate Kavan
Karam Nam Baranat Sumat ||1||

Bujang Preyat Chand

Namastang Akaley
Namastang Kripaley
Namastang Arūpey
Namastang Anūpey ||2||
Namastang Abey-key
Namastang Aley-key
Namastang Aka-ey
Namastang Aja-ey ||3||
Namastang Aganjey
Namastang Abanjey

71

Namastang Anamey
Namastang Atamey ||4||
Namastang Akaramang
Namastang Adaramang
Namastang Anamang
Namastang Adamang ||5||
Namastang Aji-tey
Namastang Abi-tey
Namastang Abahey
Namastang Adahey ||6||
Namastang Anïley
Namastang Anadey
Namastang Ache-dey
Namastang Agadey ||7||
Namastang Aganjey
Namastang Abanjey
Namastang Udarey
Namastang Aparey ||8||
Namastang Su-ekey
Namastang Ane-key
Namastang Abū-tey
Namastang Ajūpey ||9||
Namastang Nirkarmey
Namastang Nirbarmey
Namastang Nirdesey
Namastang Nirbesey ||10||
Namastang Nirnamey
Namastang Nirkamey
Namastang Nirdatey
Namastang Nirgatey ||11||
Namastang Nirdūtey
Namastang Abūtey
Namastang Alo-key
Namastang Aso-key ||12||
Namastang Nirtapey
Namastang Atapey
Namastang Tri-maney
Namastang Nidaney ||13||
Namastang Aga-hey
Namastang Aba-hey
Namastang Tri-bargey
Namastang Asargey ||14||
Namastang Prabogey
Namastang Sūjogey
Namastang Arangey
Namastang Abangey ||15||
Namastang Aganmey
Namastast Ranmey

Namastang Jalasrey
Namastang Nirasey ||16||
Namastang Ajatey
Namastang Apatey
Namastang Amajbey
Namastast Aj-bey ||17||
Namastang Ade-sey
Namastang Abe-sey
Namastang Nirdamey
Namastang Nirbamey ||18||
Namo Sarab Kaley
Namo Sarab Dia-ley
Namo Sarab Rūpey
Namo Sarab Būpey ||19||
Namo Sarab Kapey
Namo Sarab Tapey
Namo Sarab Kaley
Namo Sarab Paley ||20||
Namastast Devey
amastang Abhevey
Namastang Ajanmey
Namastang Sūbanmey ||21||
Namo Sarab Gau-ney
Namo Sarab Bau-ney
Namo Sarab Rangey
Namo Sarab Bangey ||22||
Namo Kal Kaley
Namo Sat Dia-ley
Namastang Abarney
Namastang Amarney ||23||
Namastang Jira-rang
Namastang Kirta-rang
Namo Sarab Dandey
Namo Sat Abandey ||24||
Namastang Nir-sakey
Namastang Nir-bakey
Namastang Rahimey
Namastang Karimey ||25||
Namastang Anantey
Namastang Mahantey
Namastast Ragey
Namastang Sūhagey ||26||
Namo Sarab Sokang
Namo Sarab Pokang
Namo Sarab Karta
Namo Sarab Harta ||27||
Namo Jog Jogey
Namo Bog Bogey

Namo Sarab Dialey
Namo Sarab Paley ||28||

Chachri Chand Tav Prasad

Arūp Hae Anūp Hae
Aju Hae Abu Hae ||29||
Alek Hae Abek Hae
Anam Hae Akam Hae ||30||
Adey Hae Abey Hae
Ajit Hae Abit Hae ||31||
Tirman Hae Nidan Hae
Tirbarg Hae Asarg Hae ||32||
Anil Hae Anad Hae
Ajey Hae Ajad Hae ||33||
Ajanam Hae Abarn Hae
Abūt Hae Abarn Hae ||34||
Aganj Hae Abanj Hae
Ajūj Hae Ajanj Hae ||35||
Amik Hae Rafik Hae
Adand Hae Aband Hae ||36||
Nirbūj Hae Asūj Hae
Akal Hae Ajal Hae ||37||
Alal Hae Aja Hae
Anant Hae Mahant Hae ||38||
Alik Hae Nirsrik Hae
Nirlanb Hae Asanb Hae ||39||
Agan Hae Ajan Hae
Abūt Hae Achūt Hae ||40||
Alok Hae Asok Hae
Akarm Hae Abarm Hae ||41||
Ajit Hae Abit Hae
Aba Hae Aga Hae ||42||
Aman Hae Nidan Hae
Anek Hae Fir-ek Hae ||43||

Bujang Preyat Chand

Namo Sarab Maney
Samasti Nidaney
Namo Deyv Deyv-ey
Abeki Abe-vey ||44||
Namo Kal Kaley
Namo Sarab Paley
Namo Sarag Gauney
Namo Sarag Bauney ||45||
Anangi Anathey
Nirsangi Pramatey

74

Namo Ban Baney
Namo Man Maney ||46||
Namo Chandr Chandrey
Namo Ban Baney
Namo Git Gitey
Namo Tan Taney ||47||
Namo Nrit Nritey
Namo Nad Nadey
Namo Pan Paney
Namo Bad Badey ||48||
Anangi Anamey
Samasti Sarūpey
Prabangi Pramatey
Samasti Bibūtey ||49||
Kalankang Bina-ney
Kalanki Sarūpey
Namo Raj Rajey S
warang Param Rūpey ||50||
Namo Jog Jogey
Swarang Pram Sïd-ey
Namo Raj Rajey
Swarang Param Brïdey ||51||
Namo Sastr Paney
Namo Astr Maney
Namo Param Giata
Namo Lok Mata ||52||
Abeki Abarmi
Abogi Abugtey
Namo Jog Jogey
Swarang Param Jūgtey ||53||
Namo Nït Nareney
Krur Karmey
Namo Pret Apret
Deyvey Sū-darmey ||54||
Namo Rog Harta
Namo Rag Rūpey
Namo Sa Sahang
Namo Būp Būpey ||55||
Namo Dan Daney
Namo Man Maney
Namo Rog Rogey
Namastang Sna-ney ||56||
Namo Mantr Mantrang
Namo Jantr Jantrang
Namo Isht Ishtey
Namo Tantr Tantrang ||57||
Sada Sachi-da-nang
Sarbang Pranasi

Anūpey Arūpey
Samastūl Nivasey ||58||
Sada Sïd-ïda
Būd-da Brïd Karta
Ado Urd Ardang
Agang Og Harta ||59||
Parang Param Parme
Swarang Proch Palang
Sada Sarab-da
Sïd Data Dialang ||60||
Achedi Abedi
Anamang Akamang
Samasto Paraji
Samastast Damang ||61||

Tera Jor Chachri Chand

Jaley Hae Taley Hae
Abit Hae Abey Hae ||62||
Prabu Hae Aju Hae
Ades Hae Abes Hae ||63||

Būjang Prayat Chand

Adadey Abadey
Anandi Sarūpey
Namo Sarab Maney
Samasti Nidaney ||64||
Namastang Nirnatey
Namastang Pramatey
Namastang Aganjey
Namastang Abanjey ||65||
Namastang Akaley
Namastang Apaley
Namo Sarab De-sey
Namo Sarab Be-sey ||66||
Namo Raj Rajey
Namo Saj Sajey
Namo Sha Sha-hey
Namo Mah Mahey ||67||
Namo Git Gitey
Namo Prit Pritey
Namo Rok Rokey
Namo Sok Sokey ||68||
Namo Sarab Rogey
Namo Sarab Bogey
Namo Sarab Ji-tang
Namo Sarag Bi-tang ||69||

Namo Sab Gianang
Namo Param Tanang
Namo Sarab Mantrang
Namo Sarab Jantrang ||70||
Namo Sarab Dri-sang
Namo Sarab Kri-sang
Namo Sarab Rangey
Tri-bangi Anangey ||71||
Namo Jiv Jivang
Namo Bij Bijey
Aki-jey Abi-jey
Samastang Prasi-jey ||72||
Kri-palang Sarūpey
Kū-karmang Pranasi
Sada Sarab-da
Rïd Sïdang Nivasi ||73||

Charpat Chand Tav Prasad

Amrït Karmey
Abrït Darmey
Akal Jogey
Achal Bogey ||74||
Achal Rajey
Atal Sajey
Akal Darmang
Alak Karmang ||75||
Sarbang Data
Sarbang Giata
Sarbang Baney
Sarbang Maney ||76||
Sarbang Pranang
Sarbang Tranang
Sarbang Būgta
Sarbang Jūgta ||77||
Sarbang Dey-vang
Sarbang Bey-vang
Sarbang Kaley
Sarbang Paley ||78||

Rual Chand Tav Prasad

Adi Rūpey Anad
Mūrït Ajon Purak Apar
Sarab Man Tri-man Deyv
Abeyv Adi Udar
Sarab Palak Sarab Galak
Sarab Ko Pūni Kal

Jatra Tatra Bi-raji
Avdūt Rūp Rasal ||79||
Nam Tam Na Jat
Jakar Rūp Rang Na Rek
Adi Pūrïk Udar Mūrït
Ajoni Adi Asek
Des Aur-na Bes Jakar
Rūp Rek Na Rag
Jatra Tatra Dïsa Vïsa
Hu-e Feylio Anūrag ||80||
Nam Kam Bïhïn Pekat
Dam Hūn Ney Ja-e
Sarab Nam Sarbatra
Man Sadeyv Manat Ta-e
Ek Mūrït Anek Darsan
Kïn Rūp Anek
Kel Kel Akel Kelan
Ant Ko Fir Ek ||81||
Deyv Beyv Na Jani
Je Bed Aur Kateb
Rūp Rang Na Jat
Pat Su Jani Ke Jeb
Tat Mat Na Jat Jakar
Janam Maran Bïhïn
Chakr Bakr Firey
Chatr Chak Mani Pūr Tïn ||82||
Lok Chauda Ke Bi-key
Jag Japi Je Jap
Adi Deyb Anad Mūrït Tapio
Sabey Je Tap-e
Param Rūp Pūnit Mūrït
Pūrïn Pūrk Apar
Sarab Bïsu Rachio Su-yambav
Garen Banjen-har ||83||
Kal Hin Kala San-jūgït
Akal Pūrk Ades
Daram Dam Su Baram
Ret Abūt Alek Abes
Ang Rag Na Rang
Jakey Jat Pat Na Nam
Gareb Ganjen Dūst
Banjen Mūkït Deyk Kam ||84||
Ap Rūp Amik An
Ustat Ek Pūrk Avdūt
Gareb Ganjen Sareb
Banjen Ad Rūp Asūt
Ang Hin Abang Anatam

Ek Pūrk Apar
Sarab Leyk Sarab Geyk
Sarab Ko Pratipar ||85||
Sarab Ganta Sarab Hanta
Sarab Te Anbek
Sarab Sastr Na Jani
Je Rūp Rang Ar Rek
Param Beyd Pūran
Jakey Net Bakat Nït
Kot Sin-mrït Pūrïn
Sastr Na Avi Vo Chït ||86||

Madubar Chand Tav Prasad

Gūn Gan Udar
Meyma Apar
Asan Abang
Upma Anang ||87||
Anbau Prakas
Nïsdïn Anas
Ajan Ba-u
Sahan Sau ||88||
Rajan Raj
Banan Ban
Deyvan Deyv
Upma Mahan ||89||
Indran Indr
Balan Bal
Rankan Rank
Kalan Kal ||90||
Anbūt Ang
Aba Abang
Gatï Mitï Apar
Gūn Gan Udar ||91||
Mūn Gan Pranam
Nirbey Nikam
At Dūt Prachand
Mit Gat Akand ||92||
Alïsya Karam
Adrïsya Daram
Sarba Barnadeya
Andand Badeya ||93||

Chachri Chand Tav Prasad

Gobïndey Mūkandey
Udarey Aparey ||94||

Hariang Kariang
Nirnamey Akamey ||95||

Būjang Preyat Chand

Chatra Chakra Karta
Chatra Chakra Harta
Chatra Chakra Daney
Chatra Chakra Janey ||96||
Chatra Chakra Varti
Chatra Chakra Barti
Chatra Chakra Paley
Chatra Chakra Kaley ||97||
Chatra Chakra Pasey
Chatra Chakra Vasey
Chatra Chakra Man-yey
Chatra Chakra Dan-yey ||98||

Chachri Chand

Na Satrey Na Mïtrey
Na Barmang Na Bïtrey ||99||
Na Karmang Ka-ey
Ajanmang Aj-ey ||100||
Na Chïtrey Na Mïtrey
Pare Hae Pavi-trey ||101||
Prïtï-sey Adï-sey
Adrï-sey Akrï-sey ||102||

Bagvati Chand Tav Prasad Kats-tey

Ke Achïj Desey
Ke Abij Besey
Ke Aganj Karmey
Ke Abanj Barmey ||103||
Ke Abij Lokey
Ke Adït Sokey
Ke Avdūt Barney
Ke Bïbūt Karney ||104||
Ke Rajang Praba Hae
Ke Darmang Dūja Hae
Ke Asok Barney
Ke Sarba Abarney ||105||
Ke Jagtang Krïti Hae
Ke Chatrang Chatri Hae
Ke Bramang Sarūpey
Ke Anbau Anūpe ||106||
Ke Ad Adeyv Hae

Ke Ap Abeyv Hae
Ke Chrtang Bi-hiney
Ke Ekey Adiney ||107||
Ke Rozi Razakey
Rahimey Rihakey
Ke Pak Bi-eb Hae
Ke Geybūl Geb Hae ||108||
Ke Afual Gūna Hae
Ke Shahan Sha Hae
Ke Karan Kūnïnd Hae
Ke Rozi Dïhand Hae ||109||
Ke Razak Rahim Hae
Ke Karmang Karim Hae
Ke Sarbang Kali Hae
Ke Sarbang Dali Hae ||110||
Ke Sarbatra Man-yey
Ke Sarbatra Dana-yey
Ke Sarbatra Gauney
Ke Sarbatra Bauney ||111||
Ke Sarbatra Desey
Ke Sarbatra Besey
Ke Sarbatra Rajey
Ke Sarbatra Sajey ||112||
Ke Sarbatra Diney
Ke Sarbatra Liney
Ke Sarbatra Jaho
Ke Sarbatra Baho ||113||
Ke Sarbatra Desey
Ke Sarbatra Besey
Ke Sarbatra Kaley
Ke Sarbatra Paley ||114||
Ke Sarbatra Hanta
Ke Sarbatra Ganta
Ke Sarbatra Beki
Ke Sarbatra Peki ||115||
Ke Sarbatra Kajey
Ke Sarbatra Rajey
Ke Sarbatra Sokey
Ke Sarbatra Pokey ||116||
Ke Sarbatra Traney
Ke Sarbatra Praney
Ke Sarbatra Desey
Ke Sarbatra Besey ||117||
Ke Sarbatra Mana-yey
Sadey-vang Pradana-yey
Ke Sarbatra Japa-yey
Ke Sarbatra Tapa-yey ||118||
Ke Sarbatra Baney

Ke Sarbatra Maney
Ke Sarbatra Indrey
Ke Sarbatra Chandrey ||119||
Ke Sarbang Kalimey
Ke Parmang Fahimey
Ke Akal Alamey
Ke Sahïb Kalamey ||120||
Ke Hūsnal Vaju Hae
Tamamūl Rūju Hae
Hamesūl Salamey
Salikat Mūdamey ||121||
Ganimūl Shikastey
Garibūl Prastey
Bilandūl Makaney
Zaminūl Zamaney ||122||
Tamizūl Tamamey
Rūjual Nidaney
Harifūl Azimey
Razeyk Yakiney ||123||
Anekūl Trang Hae
Abed Hae Abang Hae
Azizūl Nivaz Hae
Ganimūl Kiraj Hae ||124||
Nirūkat Sarūp Hae
Tri-mūkat Bibūt Hae
Prabūgat Praba Hae
Sūjūgat Sūda Hae ||125||
Sadey-vang Sarūp Hae
Abedi Anūp Hae
Samasto Paraj Hae
Sada Sarab Saj Hae ||126||
Samastūl Salam Hae
Sadeyvūl Akam Hae
Nirbad Sarūp Hae
Adag Hae Anūp Hae ||127||
O-ang Ad Rūpey
Anad Sarūpey
Anangi Anamey
Tri-bangi Tri-kamey ||128||
Tri-bargang Tri-Bardey
Aganjey Agad-hey
Sūbang Sarab Bagey
Su Sarba Anūragey ||129||
Tri-būgat Sarūp Hae
Achij Hae Achūt Hae
Ke Narkang Pranas Hae

Priti-ūl Pravas Hae ||130||
Nirūkat Praba Hae
adey-vang Sada Hae
Bibūgat Sarūp Hae
Prajūgat Anūp Hae ||131||
Nirūkat Sada Hae
Bibūgat Praba Hae
Anūkat Sarūp Hae
Prajūgat Anūp Hae ||132||

Chachri Chand

Abang Hae Anang Hae
Abek Hae Alek Hae ||133||
Abarm Hae Akarm Hae
Anad Hae Jūgad Hae ||134||
Ajey Hae Abai Hae
Abūt Hae Adūt Hae ||135||
Anas Hae Udas Hae
Adand Hae Aband Hae ||136||
Abagat Hae Birakat Hae
Asan Hae Prakas Hae ||137||
Nichint Hae Sūnint Hae
Alik Hae Adik Hae ||138||
Alek Hae Abek Hae
Ada Hae Aga Hae ||139||
Asanb Hae Aganb Hae
Anil Hae Anad Hae ||140||
Anit Hae Sūnit Hae
Ajat Hae Ajad Hae ||141||

Charpat Chand Tav Prasad

Sarbang Hanta Sarbang Ganta
Sarbang Kiata Sarbang Giata ||142||
Sarbang Harta Sarbang Karta
Sarbang Pranang Sarbang Tranang ||143||
Sarbang Karmang Sarbang Darmang
Sarbang Jūgta Sarbang Mūkta ||144||

Rasaval Chand Tav Prasad

Namo Narak Nasey
Sadey-vang Prakasey
Anangang Sarūpe
Abangang Bibūtey ||145||
Pramatang Pramatey

Sada Sarab Satey
Agad Sarūpey
Nirbad Bibūtey ||146||
Anangi Anamey
Tri-bangi Tri-kamey
Nirbangi Sarūpey
Sarbangi Anūpey ||147||
Na Portrey Na Pūtrey
Na Satrey Na Mitrey
Na Tatey Na Matey
Na Jatey Na Patey ||148||
Nirsakang Sarik Hae
Amito Amik Hae
Sadey-vang Praba Hae
Ajey Hae Aja Hae ||149||

Bagvati Chand Tav Prasad

Ke Zahar Zahūr Hae
Ke Hazar Hazūr Hae
Hemesūl Salam Hae
Samastal Kalam Hae ||150||
Ke Sahïb Dimag Hae
Ke Hūsal Charag Hae
Ke Kamal Karim Hae
Ke Razak Rahim Hae ||151||
Ke Rozi Dïhen Hae
Ke Razak Rahïnd Hae
Karimūl Kamal Hae
Ke Hūsnal Jamal Hae ||152||
Ganimūl Kiraj Hae
Garibūl Nivaz Hae
Harifūl Shikan Hae
Hirasūl Fikan Hae ||153||
Kalankang Pranas Hae
Samastūl Nivas Hae
Aganjūl Ganim Hae
Reza-eyk Rahim Hae ||154||
Samastūl Zūban Hae
Ke Sahïb Kiran Hae
Ke Narkang Pranas Hae
Bahishtūl Nivas Hae ||155||
Ke Sarbūl Gavan Hae
Hamesūl Ravan Hae
Tamamūl Tamiz Hae
Samastūl Aziz Hae ||156||
Parang Param Is Hae

Samastūl Adis Hae
Adesūl Alek Hae
Hamesūl Abek Hae ||157||
Zaminal Zaman Hae
Amikūl Iman Hae
Karimūl Kamal Hae
Ke Jūrt Jamal Hae ||158||
Ke Achlang Prakas Hae
Ke Amito Sūbas Hae
Ke Ajab Sarūp Hae
Ke Amito Bibūt Hae ||159||
Ke Amito Pas Hae
Ke Atam Praba Hae
Ke Achlang Anang Hae
Ke Amito Abang Hae ||160||

Madubar Chand Tav Prasad

Mūn Man Pranam
Gūn Gan Mudam
Ar Bar Aganj
Har Nar Prabanj ||161||
An Gan Pranam
Mun Man Salam
Har Nar Akand
Bar Nar Amand ||162||
Anbav Anas
Mūn Man Prakas
Gun Gan Pranam
Jal Tal Mudam ||163||
Anch-hij Ang Asan Abang
Upma Apar Gati Miti Udar ||164||
Jal Tal Amand Dïs Vïs Aband
Jal Tal Mahant Dïs Vïs Beant ||165||
Anbav Anas Drit Dar Duras
Ajan Ba Ekey Sada-a ||166||
Onkar Adi Kathni Anad
Kal Kand Kial Gurbar Akal ||167||
Gar Gar Pranam Chït Charn Nam
Anch-hij Gat Ajij Na Bat ||168||
Anj-hanj Gat Anranj Bat
Antūt Bandar Antat Apar ||169||
Adit Daram Ati Dit Karam
Anbran Anant Data Mahant ||170||

Hari Bol Mana Chand Tav Prasad

Karunal-ye Hae
Ar Gal-ye Hae
Kal Kandan Hae
Mey Mandan Hae ||171||
Jagtesvar Hae
Parmesvar Hae
Kali Karan Hae
Sarab Uburan Hae ||172||
Frit Ke Dran Hae
Jag Ke Kran Hae
Man Maneya Hae
Jag Janeya Hae ||173||
Sarbang Bar Hae
Sarbang Kar Hae
Sarab Pasiya Hae
Sarab Nasiya Hae ||174||
Karunakar Hae
Bisvanbar Hae
Sarbesvar Hae
Jagtesvar Hae ||175||
Bramandas Hae
Kal Kandas Hae
Par Te par Hae
Karunakar Hae ||176||
Ajapa Jap Hae
Atapa Tap Hae
Akrita Krit Hae
Amrita Mrit Hae ||177||
Amrita Mrit Hae
Karuna Krit Hae
Akrita Krit Hae
Darni Drit Hae ||178||
Amitesvar Hae
Parmesvar Hae
Akrita Krit Hae
Amrita Mrit Hae ||179||
Ajba Krit Hae
Amrita Mrit Hae
Nar Neyk Hae
Kal Geyk Hae ||180||
Bisvanbar Hae
Karunalya Hae
Nrip Neyk Hae
Sarab Peyk Hae ||181||
Bav Banjan Hae
Ar Ganjan Hae
Rip Tapan Hae
Jap Japan Hae ||182||

Aklang Krït Hae
Sarba Krït Hae
Karta Kar Hae
Harta Har Hae ||183||
Parmatam Hae
Sarbatam Hae
Atam Bas Hae
Jas-ke Jas Hae ||184||

Bujang Prayat Chand

Namo Surj Surjey
Namo Chandr Chandrey
Namo Raj Rajey
Namo Ïndr Ïndrey
Namo And-karey
Namo Teyj Tey-jey
Namo Brïnd Brïndey
Namo Bij Bijey ||185||
Namo Rajsang
Tamsang Sat Rūpey
Namo Pram Tatang
Ata-tang Sarūpey
Namo Jog Jogey
Namo Gian Gianey
Namo Mantr Mantrey
Namo Dian Dianey ||186||
Namo Jūd Jūdey
Namo Gian Gianey
Namo Boj Bojey
Namo Pan Paney
Namo Kala Karta
Namo Sant Rūpey
Namo Ïndr Ïndrey
Anadang Bibūtey ||187||
Kalankar Rūpey
Alankar Alankey
Namo As Asey
Namo Bank Bankey
Abangi Sarūpey
Anangi Anamey
Tribangi Trikaley
Anangi Akamey ||188||

Ek Achari Chand

Ajai Alai
Abhai Abai ||189||

87

Abū Ajū
Anas Akas ||190||
Aganj Abanj
Alak Abak ||191||
Akal Deyal
Aleyk Abeyk ||192||
Anam Akam
Agaha Adaha ||193||
Anatey Parmatey
Ajoni Amoni ||194||
Na Ragey Na Rangey
Na Rūpey Na Reykey ||195||
Akaramang Agaramang
Aganjey Aleykey ||196||

Bujang Prayat Chand

Namastūl Pranamey
Samastūl Pranasey
Aganjūl Anamey
Samastūl Nivasey
Nrikamang Bibūtey
Samastūl Sarūpey
Kūkarmang Pranasi
Sūdarmang Bibūtey ||197||
Sada Sat-chïd-anand
Satrang Pranasi
Karimūl Kūninda
Samastūl Nivasi
Aja-eyb Bibūtey
Gaja-eyb Ganimey
Hariang Kariang
Karimūl Rahimey ||198||
Chatr Chakr Varti
Chatr Chakr Būgatey
Sūyambav Sūbang
Sarab Da Sarab Jū-gatey
Dūkalang Pranasi
Dey-alang Sarūpey
Sada-ang Sangey
Abang-ang Bïbūtey ||199||

God has no mark, color, caste or lineage.
None can describe His form, complexion, outline and costume.
He is perpetual, self-illuminated, and measureless in power.
God is the King of kings and God of millions of Indras.
God is the Emperor of the three worlds, demi-gods, man and demons;

And the woods and dales proclaim Him as indescribable.
No one can tell all the Names of God,
Who is called by special Name by the wise, according to His excellences and doings. ||1||

I salute immortal God. I salute merciful God.
I salute formless God. I salute God, Who is without parallel. ||2||
I salute God, Who has no dress. I salute God, Whose portrait cannot be drawn.
I salute God, Who has no body. I salute God, Who was not born. ||3||
I salute God, Who cannot be conquered. I salute God, Who cannot be destroyed.
I salute God, Who has no particular name. I salute God, Who has no particular place. ||4||
I salute God, Who is above rituals and is not bound to do any work.
I salute God, Who is above formal observances.
I salute God, Who has no special name. I salute God, Who has no particular home. ||5||
I salute God, Who cannot be conquered. I salute God, Who is not afraid of anyone.
I salute unshakeable God. I salute God, Who cannot be overthrown. ||6||
I salute God, Who has no color or form. I salute God, Who has no beginning.
I salute God, Who cannot be broken. I salute God, Who is unfathomable. ||7||
I salute God, Who is invincible. I salute God, Who cannot be smashed.
I salute God, Who is large hearted. I salute God, Who is boundless. ||8||
I salute God, Who is One. I salute God, Who has many manifestations.
I salute God, Who is not made of five elements. I salute God, Who is free from entanglements. ||9||
I salute God, Who is above rituals and has no engagements. I salute God, Who is free from doubts.
I salute God, Who does not belong to any one region. I salute God, Who has no dress. ||10||
I salute God, Who has no particular name. I salute God, Who is desireless.
I salute God, Who is above five elements. I salute God, Who cannot be injured. ||11||
I salute God, Who is immoveable. I salute God, Who is not made of five elements.
I salute God, Who is invisible. I salute God, Who has no worries. ||12||
I salute God, Who is above all troubles. I salute God, Who cannot be installed (as a statue).
I salute God, Who is honored by the living beings of the three worlds.
I salute God, Who is the Real Treasure. ||13||
I salute God, Whose depth is unknown. I salute God, Who is unshakeable.
I salute God, Who is the Fountain of three supreme virtues; Who cannot be created. ||14||
I salute God, Who enjoys all. I salute God, who is Omnipresent.
I salute God, Who has no color. I salute God, Who cannot be destroyed. ||15||
I salute God, Who is incomprehensible. I salute God, Who is most beautiful.
I salute God, Who pervades the oceans. I salute God, Who needs no help. ||16||
I salute God, Who has no caste. I salute God, Who has no dynasty.
I salute God, Who has no religion. I salute God, Who is wonderful. ||17||
I salute God, Who does not belong to a particular country.
I salute God, Who wears no dress. I salute God, Who has no particular home.
I salute God, Who is unborn and unaffected by mammon. ||18||
I salute God, Who causes all to die. I salute God, Who showers mercy on all.
I salute God, Who is present in all beings. I salute God, Who is the Emperor of all. ||19||
I salute God, Who is the destroyer and creator of all.
I salute God, Who kills all. I salute God, Who tends all. ||20||
I salute God, Who is the Light-giving object of worship.
I salute God, Whose secrets cannot be known.
I salute God, Who is unborn. I salute God, Who is most beautiful. ||21||
I salute God, Who can reach all. I salute God, Who resides everywhere.
I salute God, Who is the creator of all colors. I salute God, Who is the destroyer of all. ||22||
I salute God, Who can destroy death itself. I salute God, Who is the fountain of mercy.
I salute God, Who is colorless and indescribable. I salute God, Who never dies. ||23||

I salute God, Who never becomes old. I salute God, Who creates all.
I salute God, Who causes all programs to be accomplished.
I salute God, Who is free from all restrictions. ||24||
I salute God, Who has no relatives. I salute God, Who is not afraid of anybody.
I salute God, Who is merciful. I salute God, Who bestows gifts. ||25||
I salute God, Who is unlimited. I salute God, Who is the biggest of all.
I salute God, Who is all love. I salute God, Who is the highest. ||26||
I salute God, Who destroys all. I salute God, Who nurses all.
I salute God, Who creates all. I salute God, Who destroys all. ||27||
I salute God, Who is the biggest Yogi. I salute God, Who is the biggest Family-man.
I salute God, Who shows mercy to all. I salute God, Who nurses all. ||28||

The Bani is uttered with God's Grace.

God has no form. God has no parallel. God is immoveable. God does not take birth. ||29||
God cannot be described. God has no dress. God has no particular name and no desires. ||30||
God is beyond comprehension of human mind. God's secrets cannot be known.
God cannot be conquered. God is not afraid of anybody. ||31||
God is worshipped in the three worlds. God is the Treasure of everything.
God is the Fountain of supreme gifts. God was never born. ||32||
God is without color; His origin is unkown. God is never old. God is not subject to births. ||33||
God was not born; has no color or caste.
God is above the elements & needs nobody to nurse Him. ||34||
God cannot be conquered or injured. None can fight with God. God is unshakeable. ||35||
God is very deep; friend of all. God is free from all entanglements and from all bondages. ||36||
None can know God as he is beyond human comprehension.
God is free from death and the reach of mammon. ||37||
God cannot be found. God has no special place. God is boundless. God is greatest of all. ||38||
Nobody can portray God. God has no relatives, needs no support and cannot be understood. ||39||
God is beyond reach, unborn. God is above five elements and cannot be touched by anybody. ||40||
God cannot be seen by human eyes. He has no worries & is beyond rites. God has no doubts. ||41||
God cannot be conquered. God has no fears.
God is steady like a mountain. God's depth cannot be known as in the case of ocean. ||42||
God cannot be measured or weighed.
God is the Treasure of everything and has countless forms. Still He has one form. ||43||

Salutations to God, Who is respected by all; Who is the treasure of everything.
Salutations to God, Who is above all gods. God has no dress and is mysterious. ||44||
Salutations to God, Who can destroy death; Who nurses all.
Salutations to God, Who can reach all places; Who is present in all places. ||45||
God, Who is Master of all, has no body. No one is equal to God.
Salutations to God, Who is the Sun of suns; Who is respected by all. ||46||
Salutations to God, Who gives light to the moon; Who gives light to the sun.
Salutations to God, Who is the Creator of songs; Who is the Creator of different tunes. ||47||
Salutations to God, Who makes others dance; Who is the Creator of sounds.
Salutations to God, Who beats the drum. Then the world drama is played. ||48||
Salutations to God, Who has no body or name; Whose beauty is present in all.
God can cause the end of creation. God is the bestower of spiritual and miraculous powers. ||49||
God is free from all blots & is pure.
Salutations to God, Who is the King of kings & highest of all. ||50||
Salutations to God, Who is the biggest Yogi and Sidh.
Salutations to God, Who is the Emperor of emperors and biggest Commander. ||51||

Salutations to God, Who weilds sword and weapons; Who can throw arrows and other weapons.
Salutations to God, Who knows everything; Who as mother, loves the world. ||52||
God has no dress and is free from all doubts, as well as temptations of worldly evils.
Salutations to God, Who is the Yogi of yogis and whose ways are supreme. ||53||
Salutations to God, Who always protects all and sets right the evil-doer with a strong hand.
Salutations to God, Who nurses the world as family, including the virtuous, evil and sprites. ||54||
Salutations to God, Who kills diseases and is the Fountain of love.
Salutations to God, Who is the Emperor of emperors. ||55||
Salutations to God, the biggest donor & Whom the most honored men pay highest respects.
Salutations to God, Who kills all diseases, restores health and washes sins. ||56||
Salutations to God, Whose Name is the biggest magical word.
Salutations to God, Whose Name is the real jantar (amulet) and tantar (charm).
God is the biggest object of worship.
God (God's Name) is the biggest tantar (charm). ||57||
God is the Fountain of truth, intelligence, peace, and pleasure and can destroy all.
None is bigger than God, Who is the cause of worldly beauties and is present everywhere. ||58||
God is the giver of Spiritual power and he confers true wisdom and success.
God is present in the nether regions, the skies, & in space; and is the destroyer of all sins. ||59||
God is the biggest Master and nurses all, without being seen.
God gives success and mental power, and is the Fountain of pity. ||60||
God cannot be harmed or destroyed by anybody and He has no name or desire.
God is the conquerer of all and is present everywhere and in all living beings. ||61||
God is present in water and on land. God cannot be terrified by anybody.
God's secrets cannot be known. ||62||
God is Master of all. God is perpetual and steady; Has no particular region or dress. ||63||
God's depth is unknown and none can stand in His way. God is the source and embodiment of joy.
Salutations to God, before Whom all bow. God is the Treasure of everything. ||64||
Salutations to God, over Whom there is no master. Salutations to God, Who can destroy all.
Salutations to God, Who cannot be defeated; Whom no harm can be caused. ||65||
Salutations to God, Whom death cannot cause harm; Who does not need any protection.
Salutations to God, Who is present in all countries; Who is present in every form. ||66||
Salutations to God, Who is the King of kings. Salutations to God, Who created the entire creation.
Salutations to God, Who is the Emperor of emperors; Who gives light to the moon. ||67||
Salutations to God, Who is the Real song; Who is the Real Love.
Salutations to God, under Whose fear earth functions; Who can cause everything to dry up. ||68||
Salutations to God, Who causes death of all living beings; Who is the Real Enjoyer of everything.
Salutations to God, Who conquers all; Who causes awe and fear in everybody. ||69||
Salutations to God, Who knows all secrets; Who has created the expanse of the world.
Salutations to God, Whose Name is the biggest magic; Whose Name is the biggest amulet. ||70||
Salutations to God, Who sees everybody and attracts all; Who is present in all the colors.
Salutations to God, Who can destroy the skies, worlds and nether-lands; Who has no body. ||71||
Salutations to God, Who is the life of all. Salutations to God Who is the Primal Seed.
None can cause any trouble to God, Who does everything and remains detached.
God confers boons on all. ||72||
God is the Fountain of pity and destroyer of sins.
God is forever the source of all spiritual and miraculous powers. ||73||

With the grace of God.

God's doings are permanent. God's Laws cannot be broken.
The world is attached to God. God is the Home of permanent joys. ||74||
The Kingdom of God is permanent. God's creation is permanent.

God's Laws are perfect. God's works are beyond comprehension. ||75||
God is the universal Giver. God knows the secrets of the minds of all.
God gives light to all. God is worshipped by all. ||76||
God is the life of all. God is the shelter for all. God is the Enjoyer of all and is attached to all. ||77||
God is worshipped by all. God knows the internal conditions of all.
God can destroy all. God nourishes all. ||78||

With the grace of God.

Limitless God existed prior to the creation; His origin is untraceable.
He does not take birth, is present everywhere, and is boundless.
All living beings bow before God, Who is the Supreme Light, worshipped in the three worlds.
God's secrets are unknown; He is the origin of all and is large hearted.
God nurses all, destroys all and causes death to all.
God is the Supreme Renouncer, the fountain of tastes & pleasures and is present everywhere. ||79||
God is not called by any particular name; He does not exist at any particular place.
He has no caste, no outlines, color or mark.
God, the Primal Creator, is present in all, possesses large heart.
God is never born, exists from the beginning and is complete in all respects.
God has no particular country, no dress, no mark, no outlines and no love for any particular thing.
God is present at every place, on every side and in every corner.
His Universal Love exists everywhere. ||80||
God has no particular name, no desires, or visible place.
All living beings ever bow before God, Who is worshipped everywhere.
God is One, yet He can be seen in innumerable forms created by Him.
God plays the world drama, creates His creation, destroys the same and then He is left alone. ||81||
The secrets of God are unknown to gods and even to the religious books.
No one can describe God, Who has no color, caste or lineage.
God is beyond births and deaths and has no parents.
Sometimes God appears in His horrible form as the Destroyer in all directions;
Living beings of the three worlds bow their heads before Him. ||82||
The Name of God is being repeated and remembered in the fourteen worlds by all the living beings.
God is the Primal and Supreme object of worship,
Whose origin cannot be traced and Who has created the entire creation.
Boundless God is the biggest power; is the source of virtues.
God is complete in all respects and present in all.
God is the Creator of the universe, He is self-created; He creates and destroys the world. ||83||
God, Who is beyond death, is all powerful, is present in all, and belongs to no particular country.
God is the Fountain of truth and virtues; is free from doubts.
God is not made of five elements, is not visible and has no particular dress.
God has no form, no body, no color, no caste and no particular name.
God destroys the ego of the proud and is the destroyer of evil doers.
He confers salvation and fulfills desires. ||84||
God is self-created and is deep beyond all descriptions; His excellences cannot be narrated.
He is unique in Himself and beyond the reach of mammon (material wealth or greed).
God smashes the pride of sinners & destroys them.
God is present since the beginning, is never born and is detached.
The boundless God has no body, no Jiv Atma (individual soul).
He cannot be destroyed, has no parallel, and is present in all.
God is capable of doing everything; He destroys all and nurses all. ||85||
God approaches all, destroys all and is distinct from all.
The religious books do not know God's form, color, or marks.

The Vedas and Puranas declare that God is the highest of all and none is like Him.
None can understand God completely even by reading the many religious books of Hindus. ||86||

With the Grace of God.

God is the treasure of countless virtues and is large-hearted. His greatness is unlimited.
His seat is perpetual. None possess as many excellences as God possesses. ||87||
God is self-illuminated, is indestructible and is ever present night and day. He is indestructible.
He controls creative forces. He is the King of kings. ||88||
God is the King of kings. God is the Sun of suns.
God is above the various gods. His praises are unlimited. ||89||
He is the King of Indra. He is the Highest of the high.
He is present with the poorest men. Death works under His command. ||90||
God is not made of five elements. God's Light is perpetual.
He cannot be measured. His excellences are countless. ||91||
Countless yogis bow before God. God is free from fear and desires.
None can bear his Light. None can minimize the Grandeur of God. ||92||
His works are automatically performed. His Law most ideal.
God is the home of all beauty. None can chastise God. ||93||

With the grace of God.

God is the Nourisher of the world. God is the Giver of salvation.
God is the biggest Donor. God is limitless. ||94||
God destroys & creates all; He has no particular name & cannot be lured by any temptation. ||95||
God creates all on all sides of the universe. God destroys all on all sides of the universe.
God showers his gifts on all sides of the universe.
God knows everything in all parts of the world. ||96||
God is present on all sides in the universe. God nurses all living beings on all sides in the universe.
God protects all living beings on all sides in the universe.
God destroys all on all sides in the universe. ||97||
God resides and is present everywhere on all sides. God is worshipped everywhere.
God bestows gifts in the whole universe on all sides. ||98||
God has no enemy. God has no friend. God has no doubt. God is not afraid of anybody. ||99||
God is free from karmas and has no body.
God is not born and does not reside in any particular place. ||100||
God's portrait cannot be made. God has no friend and is detached from all and is most pure. ||101||
God is the Master of the universe. God exists from the beginning.
God is invisible. God never becomes feeble. ||102||

The verses are uttered with the grace of God.

God's place is perpetual. God's form is indestructible.
God cannot be obtained by mere rituals. God is free from all doubts. ||103||
God's place is indivisible and permanent. God can destroy the sun.
Mammon cannot influence God. God is the source of riches and honors. ||104||
God's glory gives glory to the rulers. God is the protector of truth.
God has no worries. God is the Ornament of all. ||105||
God is the Creator of the universe. God is the bravest of the brave.
God is the most beautiful and is the biggest of all. God is the Fountain of divine knowledge. ||106||
God, Who is above gods, exists from the beginning. God is self-illuminated.
None can draw God's picture. God is the Controller of Himself. ||107||

God gives nourishment to all. God showers pity on all, and confers liberation.
God is most pure and blotless. God is Invisible. ||108||
God forgives sins and is the King of kings. God is the Doer of all; gives nourishment to all. ||109||
God nurses all and takes pity. God showers His gifts.
God is the Owner of all powers. God is the Destroyer of all. ||110||
God is worshipped everywhere. God showers His gifts on all at all places.
God reaches all places. God is present in all the worlds. ||111||
God is present at every place in every country. God is manifested in all places in different dresses.
God is the King of His creation. God gives glory to all. ||112||
God confers gifts on all at all places. God is present everywhere.
God's glory exists at all places. God's Light spreads everywhere. ||113||
God exists in the universe. God is present in various dresses in the world.
God is the Killer of all at all places. God protects all at all places. ||114||
God destroys all at all places. God can reach all places.
God manifests Himself in different forms throughout.
God takes care of all the human beings at all the places. ||115||
All works are done everywhere at the instance of God.
He is present everywhere as the Supreme King.
He causes destruction everywhere. He nurses all at all places. ||116||
God's power works at all places. God is the universal life giver.
God is present at every place in every country and can be seen in various dresses in the world. ||117||
God is worshipped at all places. God is the Supreme Controller of the universe.
God is remembered everywhere. God is present everywhere. ||118||
God gives light to the sun. God is worshipped everywhere.
God is the King of the universe. God gives light to the moon. ||119||
God sits within living beings and utters sweet words. God possesses the Supreme Wisdom.
God is the Fountain of learning. God is the Creator of languages. ||120||
God is the embodiment of beauty. All look towards God.
God will exist forever. None can diminish the ever-lasting beauty of God's creation. ||121||
God can cause defeat of sinful enemies. God nurses and protects the innocent poor persons.
God's place is the highest. God is present in the world at all times. ||122||
God knows all (about the sinners, as well as the virtuous). God takes care of all. ||123||
The world is like countless waves emanating from God (Who is like the biggest ocean).
No one can know God's secrets, Who cannot be destroyed.
God protects the true devotees. God punishes the evil doers. ||124||
No one can make a portrait of God.
Whose glory is beyond mammon's reach. All living beings enjoy the Light of God.
God is the Supreme Nectar, which is present in the living beings & can be enjoyed by them. ||125||
God exists perpetually and has no rival. God, the Creator of the entire universe conquers all. ||126||
God is worshipped by all. God never has any desire.
None can stand in the way of God. God is very deep and none is equal to Him. ||127||
God is the Soul of all living beings. God existed since long before creation.
God has no body and name. God fulfills the wishes of all in the three worlds. ||128||
God is the Treasure and Controller of all things. God cannot be conquered and is very deep.
God in all forms is very beautiful. God loves all. ||129||
Living beings in all three worlds, get joys from God. God never becomes old & cannot be touched.
God can destroy hell. God is present everywhere in the universe. ||130||
God's glory cannot be depicted. God is ever present.
All get joy from God. Limitless God is without parallel and is present in all. ||131||
None can describe the form of God. All living beings enjoy the Light of God.
God's form cannot be described. God is united with everyone and is matchless. ||132||

God is indestructible. He has no limb. He has no desires. He is beyond description. ||133||
He has no doubts, is beyond rituals. He has no beginning & existed even before ages began. ||134||
He cannot be conquered. He cannot be destroyed.
He is separate from the five elements. He is unshakeable and is not afraid of anybody. ||135||
He is perpetual. He is not entangled in love for anybody.
He is not involved in any entanglements. He is beyond all restraints. ||136||
He is indifferent to love and cannot be divided.
He has no attachment for material things. He is beyond death. He is the Supreme Light. ||137||
He is carefree. He ever continues to exist. He cannot be depicted. He is invisible. ||138||
None can make His portrait; he has no custumes. He cannot be conquered & is most deep. ||139||
He is incomprehensible. He is beyond reach. He has no color. His origin is unknown. ||140||
He is unique, extraordinary and has been existing for ever. He is beyond births; fully free. ||141||

By the grace of God.

God can kill all. He can reach all. He is well known to all. He knows all. ||142||
He destroys all. He creates all. He is the Giver of life to all. He gives power to all. ||143||
He causes all things to be done. He gives virtues to all.
He is present in all. (At the same time) He is separate from all. ||144||

By the grace of God.

I bow to God, Who gives liberation from hell.
His Light is perpetual. He has got no limbs, no bodily form. His Light never fades. ||145||
He destroys those, who cause pain to others.
He accompanies all. He is Boundless. No one can stop his Light. ||146||
God has no body and no special name.
He is the Cherisher & Destroyer of three worlds. He cannot be destroyed; None is like Him. ||147||
He has no son or grandson. He has neither enemy nor friend.
He has neither father or mother. He has neither any caste nor any dynasty. ||184||
He has no relatives or collateral. He and His depth cannot be measured.
His Light is continuous. He cannot be defeated and is beyond birth. ||149||

By the grace of God.

His Light is visible. He is present everywhere. He is perpetual. Everyone sings His virtues. ||150||
He is most intelligent. He is the Fountain of Beauty and Light.
He is most merciful to all. He takes pity and gives sustenance to all. ||151||
He gives food to all. He can confer salvation. He is most bountiful. He is most beautiful. ||152||
He overpowers enemies and is the Cherisher of the poor. He destroys enemies and fear. ||153||
He removes curses, lives in all and enemies cannot win. He gives sustenance, shows pity. ||154||
God is the tongue of all (speaks within all). He is most grand.
He can destroy hell. He resides in heavens. ||155||
He reaches all. He is the Source of all pleasures. He keeps all in view. All love Him. ||156||
He is the Lord of lords. He is the Lord of all at all times.
He has no particular residence; none can make His portrait. He has no particular dress. ||157||
He is present on earth and heaven. God's mystery (religion) is deep.
His bounties are wonderful. He is the embodiment of beauty and boldness. ||158||
His Light is perpetual. His smell is most pleasant.
His beauty is wonderful. His grandeur is beyond measures. ||159||
He spreads everywhere. He is the Light of all lights.
He is ever steady and has got no body. He is boundless and imperishable. ||160||

With the grace of God.

Holy saints bow before God with devotion. He is the Treasure of limitless virtues.
Enemies, howsoever strong, cannot defeat Him. He is the lord of all men and can destroy all. ||161||
Countless living beings salute God. Saints worship Him in their minds.
God is the Emperor of mortals. God is complete in all respects. ||162||
Indestructible God is the Fountain of self created knowledge. God's Light shines within the saints.
Salutations to God, Who has countless virtues.
Salutations to God, Who is ever present in water and on land. ||163||
God never becomes old. God's seat is perpetual.
None is equal to God. None can describe the greatness of God. ||164||
God, the most beautiful, is present on waters and on lands.
God is present in every nook and corner, free from slander.
God is Supreme on lands and seas. God is present in countless forms on all sides. ||165||
Indestructible God is the Fountain of self created knowledge. God is the Lord of all on earth.
God is the only Controller of the means of creation. God is ever only One. ||166||
God is present without change everywhere. None can know God's origin through discourses.
God destroys mean enemies in an instant. God is the most powerful and immortal. ||167||
God is respected in every house. God's holy feet and name reside in every heart.
God's body never becomes old. God does not depend on anybody for anything. ||168||
God is ever steady. God's acts are free from anger.
God's stores are inexhaustible. Limitless God has not been created by anybody. ||169||
The working of God's Laws cannot be perceived. God's works are performed fearlessly.
None can injure Limitless God. God is the biggest Donor. ||170||

With the grace of God.

God is the Home of mercy. God is the Destroyer of enemies.
God is the Killer of evil doers. God gives beauty to the earth. ||171||
God is the Owner of the universe. God is the Supreme Master of all.
Wars start at the command of God. God saves all. ||172||
God is the Support of the earth. God is the Maker of the universe.
All worship God in their hearts. All try to know God. ||173||
God nourishes all. God creates all. God is close to all. God destroys all. ||174||
God is the Fountain of pity. God nurses the world.
God is the Master of all. God is the Owner of the universe. ||175||
God is the Lord of the universe. God is the Destroyer of enemies.
God is the biggest of all. God is the Fountain of pity. ||176||
God cannot be controlled by charms. God cannot be installed as an object of worship in temples.
God's statue cannot be made. God is ever immortal and is the Fountain of Nectar. ||177||
God is ever immortal and is the Fountain of Nectar. God is the Fountain of mercy.
God's image cannot be made. God is the Supporter of the earth. ||178||
God is the Owner of Nectar. God is the biggest Lord of all.
God's image cannot be made. God is ever Immortal and is the Fountain of Nectar. ||179||
God's form is wonderful. God is ever Immortal and is the Fountain of Nectar.
God is the Master of men. God is the Destroyer of enemies. ||180||
God nurses the world. God is the Home of mercy.
God is the Master of kings. God is the protector of all. ||181||
God destroys the fetters of transmigration. God conquers enemies.
God teaches lessons to enemies. God makes others to repeat His name. ||182||
God is free from blemishes. God is complete in every respect.

God is the Creator of Brahma. God is the Destroyer of Shiva. ||183||
God is the Primal Soul. All souls originate from God's Soul.
God is the Controller of Himself. God's glory surpasses all glories. ||184||

Salutations to God, Who gives Light to the sun and moon.
Salutations to God, Who is the King of Indra.
Salutations to God, Who creates pitch darkness and also the most brilliant light.
Salutations to God, Who is the biggest of all the groups of living beings and the most subtle. ||185||

Salutations to God, Who has created the quality, called Rajo gun (from which worldly love and pride originate-Rajas Guna); the quality, called Tamo gun (from which the darkness of mind originates-Tamas Guna) and the quality, called the Sato gun (from which peace originates-Satva Guna).

Salutations to God, Who is the Primal Soul and is above the five elements.
Salutations to God, Who is the Fountain of all yogas and knowledge.
Salutations to God, the biggest magic; Whose meditation is the highest form of meditation. ||186||
Salutations to God, Who conquers enemies in war, Who is the Fountain of the highest knowledge.
Salutations to God, Who infuses energy in food and drinking water, for preserving bodies.
Salutations to God, Who is the King of gods and source of whose grandeur is uknown. ||187||
Salutations to God, Who is flawless and Who gives beauty to beautiful things.
Salutations to God, the Fulfiller of hopes, Who is most beautiful.
God has no body, is indestructible and His names are many.
God can destroy the sky, the earth and the nether worlds;
His existence is perpetual and He is without body or desires. ||188||

God is Invincible. God is Indestructible. God is Fearless. God is Immortal. ||189||
God was never born. God is Perpetual. God is Indestructible. God pervades everywhere. ||190||
God is Invincible. God is Impartible. God cannot be seen. God has no hunger wants. ||191||
God is Immortal, the Home of mercy. God's portrait cannot be drawn. God has no dress. ||192||
God has no particular name and no desires. God is Unfathomable. God cannot be damaged. ||193||
God has no master and can destroy all. God is free from samskara and observes not silence. ||194||
God is above love. God has no color. God has no form. God has no tomb. ||195||
God is above bad or good deeds. God is free from doubts.
God cannot be conquered. None can draw a picture of God. ||196||

Salutations to Respected God; Who is the Destroyer of all.
Salutations to God, Who is Invincible; Who has no particular name and lives in all living beings.
Salutations to God, Whose grandeur is unaffected by any desire and can be seen in all living things.
God is the Destroyer of sins and His works are regulated according to His Laws. ||197||
God is the living source of knowledge and joy, and kills foes.
God bestows favors, creates and resides in all.
God's grandeur is wonderful and He can cause havoc on foes.
God can destroy and create; and can confer gifts and pity on all. ||198||
God is present on all sides and by His Order controls all the world.
God's Light is automatic; He is beautiful and is ever present in all living beings.
God destroys the pains of births and deaths, and is the embodiment of mercy.
God is present with all and His grandeur will never vanish. ||199||[151]

TAV PRASAD SVAYE

This short hymn from Guru Gobind Singh is merely 10 stanzas. Like *Jap Sahib*, this *bani* also appears in *Dasam Granth* (Book of the Tenth Emperor).

Ik Ong Kar Wahe Guru Ji Ki Fateh Patsahi Dasvin

Tav Prasad Svaye

Sravag sūd samu sedan ke
Dek firio gar jog jati ke

Sur surardan sūd sūdadïk
Sant sanu anek mati ke
Sarey hi deys ko dek rayo mat
Ko na dekiat Pranpati ke

Sri Bagavan ki bae kripa hu te
Ek rati bïn ek rati ke ||1||

Matey matang jare jar sang
Anūp utang surang savarey
Koti turang kurang se kūdat
Paun ke gaun kau jat nivarey
Bari būjan ke būp bali bid
Niavat sïs na jat bicharey
Ete bae tu kaha bae būpat
ant kau nangey hi pae padarey ||2||

Jit firay sab des disan ko
Bajat dol mrïdang nagarey
Gunjat gur gajan ke sundar
Hirisat hae heyraj hajarey
Būt bavïk bavan ke būpat
Kaun ganey nahïn jat bicharey
Sri pat Sri Bagvan bajey bïn
Ant kau ant ke dam sidarey ||3||

Tirath nan deya dam dan
Su sanjam nem anek bïsek-he
Bed puran ketab kuran
Jamin jaman saban ke peyk-he
Paun ahar jati jat dar
Sabey su bichar hajar-ek deyk-he
Sri Bagvan bajey, bïn būpat
Ek rati bïn ek na leyk-he ||4||

Sūd sipa Durant dūba
Su saj sana-ha durjan dalengey
Bari gūman barey man mae
Kar parbat pank haley na halengey
Tor arin maror mavasan
Matey matangan man malengey
Sri pat Sri Bagvan kripa bïn
Tiag jahan nidan chalengey ||5||

Bir apar badey bariar
Abicharey sar ki dar bacheya
Torat deys malïnd mavasan
Matey gajan ke man maleya
Garey garan ke toran har
Su batan hi chak char laveya
Saib sri sab ko sir na-ik
Jachak anek su-ek dïveya ||6||
Danav deyv fanïnd nïsachar
Būt bavïk bavan japen-gey
Jiv jitey jal mey tal mey
Pal hi pal mey sab tap tapen-gey
Pūn pratapan bad jeyt dūn
Papan ke ba-hu panj kapen-gey
Sad samu prasan fïrey jag
Satr sabey avlok chapen-gey ||7||

Manav ïndr gajïndr naradap
Jaun trïlok ko raj karen-gey
Kot snan gajadik dan
Anek suanbar saj baren-gey
Bram mahesar bisan sachipat
Ant fasey jam fas paren-gey
Je nar sri pat ke pras hae pag
Te nar fer na de daren-gey ||8||

Kaha beyo jo do lochan mūnd key
Bet rai-o bak dian lagai-o
Nat firio li-ey sat samundran
Lok geyo perlok gavai-o
Bas kio bïkian so bet-key
Asey he asey su beys bïtai-o
Sach keo sūn leyo sabey
Jïn prema kio tïn hi prab pai-o ||9||

Kahūn ley pahan pūj Dario sir
Kahūn ley lïng garey latkai-o
Kahūn lakio har avachi disa mey

Kahu pacha ko sis nïvai-o
Ko būtan ko pūjat hey pas
Ko mirtan ko pūjan dai-o
Kur kriya urjio sab hi jag
Sri Bagvan ko beyd na pay-o ||10||

The creation and creator are one. Victory is of God. Hymn from the Tenth Guru.

With the grace of God

I have seen many abodes where groups of Sarogis, Sudhs, Sidhs, Yogis & Jains reside. (I have also seen) various groups of the brave men, demons & gods, who drink nectar, & other saints, belonging to various sects.
All the ideologies of all the countries have been studied but the Lord of souls is still unseen.
All these are worthless, if these men do not earn the Grace and Love of The Lord. ||1||

If tall, valuable elephants painted in bright colors, adorned with gold are possessed.
If millions of horses, capable of fleeing at a speed faster than the wind and bounding like deer are possessed.
If countless kings, with strong arms were to visit and bow their heads;
It matters not if such powerful emperors exist because they depart naked in the end. ||2||

If they were to march and conquer all the countries beating all kinds of drums;
If herds of many beautiful elephants were to trumpet loudly & if thousands of horses of royal breed were to neigh;
Such emperors whether past, present or future, cannot be counted by anyone;
Without worshipping the Name of the Lord; they must go to their final home (of death) empty handed. ||3||

They may take baths at places of pilgrimage, exercise acts of mercy, control their passion, perform acts of charity, practice continence and perform many rituals.
They may study the Vedas, the Puranas, the Holy Quran and other books of the religions of all times, countries and places;
They may live only on the air and practice continence and thousands of such other abilities;
Even then all these methods are worthless and of no account, without the meditation upon the Love of the Lord. ||4||

If fully trained, powerful and invinceable soldiers, wearing coats of armor, were capable of crushing the enemies;
If they are confident that the mountain may move from its position by acquiring wings but their steps cannot turn back upon the battle field;
If they break the necks of their enemies and smash the pride of even the furious elephants;
They will depart from this world empty handed without receiving the blessing of God. ||5||

Many invincible and brave soldiers are capable of facing the edge of the sword without hesitation;
Even if they were to conquer many countries and subjugate the rebels and crush the furious elephants;
If they were to seize strong forts and win the whole world simply by giving threats;
God alone is the Giver & the Commander of all, Lord of all who are beggars before Him. ||6||

Demons, gods, king cobras & sprites have been reciting the Lord's name in the past and will in the future;
God can create all living things both on land and in the water in a single moment;
They earn appreciation and glory as the result of their virtuous deeds, which will destroy their past sins;
The noble saints who worship God wander the earth with joy while their enemies are cowed down on seeing them. ||7||

Men who own powerful elephants, become emperors, and rule the world;
They perform numerous ablutions and have distributed numerous elephants, and other animals, as charity and wed brides at Savambras (marriage functions);
Of all such persons, even Brahma, Vishnu, Shiva and Indra have to die at last;
Only those who fall at the feet of God will not pass through the cycles of birth & death. ||8||

What is the use of sitting with the eyes closed, feigning to meditate, like a crane?
Even those who make ablutions at the seven seas lose this world, as well as the next, without worshipping God;
Those who spend their lives doing evil deeds waste their lives in vain;
All should listen to this truth: only those who love God can realize him. ||9||

Some worship stones by bowing to them and others wear lingams around their necks;
Some claim to see God in the South and some bow their heads to the West;
Some foolishly worship idols while others adore the dead;
The whole world is busy in false ceremonies and has yet to know God's secrets. ||10||[152]

ANAND SAHIB

This Sikh Morning Prayer was composed by the Third Guru, Amar Das. It is believed that chanting this *bani* daily with unwavering concentration and dedication will result in complete happiness. Guru Amar Das describes with great detail the feelings of Supreme Bliss having discovered the True Guru. **Anand** means bliss; **Sahib** is song. *Anand Sahib* is the *song of bliss.*

Here is a story about the origin of this prayer:

There once was a Yogi who honestly meditated with as much devotion as he could. This yogi had been searching for God for a long time. In his intuition he trusted that this Guru Amar Das was a divine teacher. The Yogi was getting very old and his life on this earth was coming to an end. One day the Yogi decided to go see Guru Amar Das. After showing great respect to the Guru he said, "O Guru, ever since I heard about you, I have longed to see you. Today I am blessed to have my longing fulfilled. I have eaten little and have done a lot of yoga, yet still I have not found peace. When I leave my body I want to be reborn into your family."

Guru ji said, "Happiness and peace are not found by not eating and trying to be the best yogi, but by loving God and singing His praises. You shall be reborn into my family." The yogi made one last prayer to God and left his body.

The Guru's younger son's name was Mohri. In time Mohri's wife gave birth to a baby boy. The baby, the grandson of the Guru, was the soul of the Yogi! Guru Amar Das ji gently held the baby in his lap. He said, "His name will be Anand" Anand means 'Bliss.' The Guru began to sing a new song: "Oh, my mother Anand has come, now I'm with the True Guru....." He kept singing this beautiful song. He sang the whole Anand Sahib for the very first time. This Anand Sahib, was created in honor of the Yogi who wanted with all his heart to be in the Guru's family. It tells us how to live life full of joy. [153]

Ramkali Mehla Tija (3) Anand

Ek ong kar Satïgur prasad

Anand bai-a meyri mai
Satïguru mey pai-a
Satïgur ta pa-ia sahej
Seyti man vaji-a vadha-ia
Rag ratan parvar
Pari-a shabd gavana-ia
Shabdo ta gavaho
Hari keyra man jïni vasa-ia

Kahey Nanïk anand hoa
Satïguru mey pa-ia ||1||

Ay man meyri-a tu
Sada rahu har naley
Har nal rahu tu man
Mey-rey dūkh sab visarna
Angikar oh karey teyra
Karaj sab savarna
Sabna gala samrat su-ami
So ki-o manhu visarey
Kahey Nanïk man mey-rey
Sada rahu har naley ||2||

Sachey sahïba kia
Nahi gar tey-rey
Gar ta tey-rey sab kïch
Hey jïs deh so pavey
Sada sïfat sala teyri
Nam man vasava-ey
Nam jïn key man vasia
Vajey shabd ganey-rey
Kahey Nanïk sachey sahïb
Kia nahi gar tey-rey ||3||

Sacha Nam meyra adharo
Sach Nam adhar meyra
Jïn bhuka sab gava-ia
Kar sat sūk mana-ey
Vasi-a jïn icha sab puja-ia
Sada kurban kita Guru
Vitahu jïs dia-eyhi vadia-ia
Kahey Nanïk sūnu s
Antahu shabd darahu pi-aro
Sacha Nam meyra adharo ||4||

Vajey panch shabd tït gar sabagey
Gar sabagey shabd vajey
Kala jït gar Daria
Panch dūt tūd vas kitey
kal kantak maria
Dhur karam pa-ia tūd jïn
Ka-o se nam har key lagey
Kahey Nanïk ta sūk hoa
Tït gar anad vajey ||5||

Sachi lïvey bïn dey nimani
Dey nimani lïvey bajahu

103

Kia karey veycharia
Tūd baj samrat ko-ey
Nahi kirpa kar banvaria
Eys na-o hor ta-o nahi
Shabd lag savaria
Kahey Nanïk livey bajahu
Kia karey veycharia ||6||

Anand anand sab ko kahey
Nand guru tey jania
Jania anand sada Gur tey
Kirpa karey pi-aria
Kar kirpa kïlvïk katey
Gian anjan saria
Andrau jïn ka mo tūta tïn
Ka shabd sachey savaria
Kahey Nanïk ayu anand hey
Anand Gur tey jania ||7||

Baba jïs tu de so-i jan pavey
Pavey ta so jan de jïs no
Hor kia karahi veycharia
Ek baram buley firey da
Dïs ek nam lag savaria
Gur parsadi man ba-ia
Nirmal jïna bana bav-ey
Kahey Nanïk jïs de
Pi-arey so-i jan pav-ey ||8||

Avu sant pi-ario
Akat ki kara kahni
Kara kahni akat keyri
Kït duarey pai-ey
Tan man dan sab sa-ūp Gur
Ka-o hūkam mani-ey pai-ey
Hūkam manihu Guru keyra
Gavu sachi bani
Kahey Nanïk sanu santahu
kati-u akat kahani ||9||

Ey man chanchla chatura-i kïney na pa-ia
Chatura-i na pa-ia kïney tu sūn man meyria
Ey ma-ia moni jïn eyt baram bula-ia
Ma-ia ta moni tïney ki-ti jïn taguli pa-ia
Kurban kita tïsey vïtau jïn mo mita la-ia
Kahey Nanïk man chanchal
Chatura-i kïney na pa-ia ||10||

104

Ey man pi-aria tu sada sach samaley
Eyu kūtamb tu je deyk da chaley nahi tey-rey naley
Sat tey-rey chaley nahi tïs nal ki-o chït lai-ey
Eysa kam mūley na kichey jït ant pachota-i-ey
Satïguru ka ūpdeys sūn tu hovey tey-rey naley
Kahey Nanïk man pi-arey tu sada sach samaley ||11||

Agam agochara teyra ant na pai-a
Anto na pai-a kïney teyra apna ap tu janhey
Jia jant sab keyl teyra kia ko ak vakana-ey
Akahi ta vey-key sab tu-hey jïn jagat upa-ia
Kahey Nanïk tu sada agam hey teyra ant na pa-ia ||12||

Sur nar mūn jan amrït koj-dey so amrït Gur tey pai-a
Pai-a amrït Gur kirpa ki-ni sacha man vasa-ia
Jia jant sab tūd upa-ey ek veyk parsana-ia
Lab lob ahankar chuka Satïguru bala ba-ia
Kahey Nanïk jïs no ap tūta tïn amrït Gur tey pa-ia ||13||

Bagta ki chal nirali
Chala nirali bhagta keyri bikam marag chalna
Lab lob ahankar taj tarisna bahūt na-i bolna
Kani-ahu tïki valau nïki eyt marag jana
Gur parsadi jïni ap tajia har vasna samani
Kahey Nanïk chal bagta jūgau jūg nirali ||14||

Jio tu chala-ïhi tïv chala su-ami hor kia jana gūn tey-rey
Jiv tu chala-ïhi tïvey chala jïna marg pavey
Kar kirpa jïn nam la-ïhi se Har Har sada di-avey
Jïs no kata sūna-ïhi apni se gurdu-arey sūk pavey
Kahey Nanïk sachey sahïb jio bavey tïvey chalava-hey ||15||

Eyhu sohila shabd suhava
Shabdo suhava sada sohila Satïguru sūna-ia
Eyhu tïn key man vasia jïn darau lïkia a-ia
Ek fïrey ganey-rey karai gala gali kïney na pa-ia
Kahey Nanïk shabd sohila Satïguru sūna-ia ||16||

Pavït ho-ey sey jana jïni har dia-ia
Har dia-ia pavït ho-ey gurmūk jïni dia-ia
Pavït mata pït kūtamb sahit sio pavït sangat saba-ia
Kadey pavït sūndey pavït sey pavït jïni man vasa-ia
Kahey Nanïk sey pavït jïni gurmūk Har Har dia-ia ||17||

Karmi sahj na ūpjey vïn sajey sasa na jai
Na jai sasa kïtey sanjam rahey karam kama-ey
Sasey jio malin hey kït sanjam dota jai

105

Man dovau shabd lagau har sio rau chït la-ey
Kahey Nanïk Gur parsadi sahj ūpjey ïh sasa ïv jai ||18||

Ji-au meyley barau nirmal
Barau nirmal ji-au ta meyley tïni janam ju-ey Haria
Ey tïsna vada rog laga maran manu visaria
Veyda me nam utam so sūne nahi firey jio beytalia
Kahey Nanïk jïn sach tajia kūrey lagey tïni janam ju-ey Haria ||19||

Ji-au nirmal barau nirmal
Barau ta nirmal ji-au nirmal Satïgur tey karni kamani
Kūr ki so-ey pochey nahi mansa sach samani
Janam ratan jïni katia baley sey vanjarey
Kahey Nanïk jïn man nirmal sada reh Gur naley ||20||

Jey ko sïk Guru seyti sanmūk hovey
Hovey ta sanmūk sïk ko-i ji-au rahey Gur naley
Gur key charn hirdey dia-ey antar atmey samaley
Ap chad sada rahey parney Gur bïn avar na janey ko-ey
Kahey Nanïk sūnhu santau so sïk sanmūk ho-ey ||21||

Jey ko Gur tey veymūk hovey bïn Satïgur mūkat na pavey
Pavey mūkat na hor tey ko-i pūchau bïbey kia jai
Aneyk jūni barm avey vïn Satïgur mūkat na pa-ey
Fir mūkat pa-ey lag charni Satïguru shabd sūna-ey
Kahey Nanïk vichar deyku vïn Satïgur mūkat na pa-ey ||22||

Avu sïk Satïguru key pi-ario gavu sachi bani
Bani ta gavu Guru keyri bania sir bani
Jïn ka-o nadr karam hovey hirdey tïna samani
Pivu amrït sada rau Har rang japi-u sarïgpani
Kahey Nanïk sada gavo-ey sachi bani ||23||

Satïguru bïna hor kachi hey bani
Bani ta kachi Satïguru bajhau hor kachi bani
Kadey kachey sūndey kachey kachi ak vakani
Har Har nït karai rasna kahia kachu na jani
Chït jïn ka hir la-ia ma-ia bolan pa-ey ravani
Kahey Nanïk Satïguru bajhau hor kachi bani ||24||

Gur ka shabd ratan hey hi-rey jït jarao
Shabd ratan jït man laga eyu hoa samao
Shabd seyti man mïlia sachey la-ia bao
Apey hi-ra ratan apey jïs no dey-ey buja-ey
Kahey Nanïk shabd ratan hey hi-ra jït jarao ||25||

Sïv sakat ap upa-ey key karta apey hūkam varta-ey

Hūkam varta-ey ap vey-key gurmūk kïsey buja-ey
Torhey bandan hovey mūkat shabd man vasa-ey
Gurmūk jïs no ap karey so hovey eykas sio lïv la-ey
Kahey Nanïk ap karta apey hūkam buja-ey ||26||

Sïmrït sastar pūn pap bi-chardey tatey sar na jani
Tatey sar na janey Guru bajau tatey sar na jani
Tïhi gūni sansar baram sūta sūtia reyn viani
Gur kirpa tey sey jan jagey jina har man vasia bole amrït bani
Kahey Nanïk sotat pa-ey jïsno
Andïn harlïv lagey jagat ren-viani ||27||

Mata key udar meh partïpal karey so kio manu visari-ey
Mano kio visarey evad data, je agan meh ahar pochav-ey
Os no kihu poi na saki jïs nao apni lïv lavey
Apni lïv apey la-ey gurmūk sada samali-ey
Kahey Nanïk eyvad data so kio manu visari-ey ||28||

Jeysi agan udar meh teysi bahar ma-ia
Ma-ia agan sab iko jeyhi kartey keyl racha-ia
Ja tïs bana ta jamia parvar bala ba-ia
Lïv churki lagi tarisna ma-ia amar varta-ia
Eyh ma-ia jït har vïsrey mo ūpjey bhao dūja la-ia
Kahey Nanïk Gur parsadi jïna lïv lagi tïni vichey ma-ia pa-ia ||29||

Har ap amūlak hey mūl na pa-ia ja-ey
Mūl na pa-ia ja-ey kïsey vitau rahey lok vila-ey
Eysa Satïgur jey mïley tïs no sir sa-ūpi-ey vichau ap jai
Jïs da jio tïs mïl rahey har vasey mana-ey
Har ap amūlak hey bag tïna key nanka jïn har paley pa-ey ||30||

Har ras meyri man vanjara
Har ras meyri man vanjara Satïgur tey ras jani
Har Har nït japiu ji-au laha katiu dihari
Eyu dan tïna mïlia jïn Har apey bana
Kahey Nanïk Har ras meyri man hoa vanjara ||31||

Ey rasna tū an ras rach ra-i teyri pias na jai
Pias na jai hort kïtey jichar Har ras paley na pa-ey
Har ras pa-ey paley pi-ey Har ras ba-ur na tarisna lagey a-ey
Eyu Har ras karmi pai-ey Satïgur mïley jïsa-ey
Kahey Nanïk hor an ras sab vi-sarey ja Har vasey mana-ey ||32||
Ey sarira meyria Har tam meh jot raki ta tu jag meh a-ia
Har jot raki tūd vïch ta tu jag meh a-ia
Har apey mata apey pïta jïn jio ūpaey jagat dïka-ia
Gur parsadi būjia ta chalat hoa chalat nadïr a-ia
Kahey Nanïk sarisat ka mūl

Rachia jot rakhi ta tu jag meh a-ia ||33||

Man chao bha-ia parb agam sūnia
Har mangal ga-o saki gariu mandar bania
Har ga-o mangal nït saki-ey sog dūk na viapa-ey
Gur charn lagey dïn sabagey apna pir japey
Anahat bani Gur shabd jani Har nam Har ras bogo
Kahey Nanïk parb ap mïlia karn karan jogo ||34||

Ey sarira meyria is jag meh a-ey key kia tūd karam kama-ia
Ke karam kama-ia tūd sarira ja tu jag meh a-ia
Jïn Har teyra rachan rachia so Har man na vasa-ia
Gur parsadi Har man vasia purab lïkia pa-ia
Kahey Nanïk eyu sarir parvan hoa jïn Satïgur sio chït la-ia ||35||

Ey neytaro meyrio Har tūm meh
Jot dari Har bïn avar na deyku ko-i
Har bïn avar na deyku ko-i nadri Har nia-lia
Eyu vïs sansar tūm deyk dey
Eyu Har ka rūp hey har rūp nadri a-ia
Gur parsadi būjia ja veyka Har ek hey Har bïn avar na ko-i
Kahey Nanïk ey neytar and sey
Satïgur mïli-ey dïb darisat ho-i ||36||

Ey sarvanu meyrio sachey sūney no pata-ey
Sachey sūney no pata-ey sarir la-ey sūnu sat bani
Jït sūni man tan Haria hoa rasna ras samani
Sach alak vïdani ta ki gat kahi na jai
Kahey Nanïk amrït namsūnu
Pavitar hovu sachey sūney nopata-ey ||37||

Har jio gūfa andar rak key vaja pavan vaja-ia
Vaja-ia vaja paun nao duarey
Pargat ki-ey dasva gūpït raka-ia
Gurdu-arey la-ey bavni ekna dasva duar dïka-ia
Ta aneyk rūp nao nav nïd tïs da ant na jai pa-ia
Kahey Nanïk Har piarey-jio
Gūfandar rak key vaja pavan vaja-ia ||38||

Eyu sacha sohila sachey gar gavu
Gavu ta sohila gar sachey jïtey sada sach diavey
Sacho dia-vey ja tūd bavey gurmūk jïna būjavey
Ih sach sabna ka kasam hey jïs baksey so jan pavey
Kahey Nanïk sach sohila sachey gar gavey ||39||

Anad sūnu vad-bagio sagal manorath pūrey
Parbarm parab pa-ia ūtrey sagal visūrey

Dūk rog santap ūtrey sūni sachi bani
Sant sajan ba-ey sarsey pūrey Gur tey jani
Sūntey pūnit katey pavït Satïgur rahia barpurey
Bïnvant Nanïk Gur charn lagey vajey anad tūrey ||40||1||

Song of Bliss
From the Third Guru

One Creator of the One Creation. By The Grace Of The True Guru:
I am in ecstasy, O my Mother, for I have found my True Guru.
I have found the True Guru, with intuitive ease, and my mind vibrates with the music of bliss.
The jewelled melodies & their celestial harmonies have come to sing the Word of the Shabd.
The Lord dwells within the minds of those who sing the Shabd.
Says Nanak, I am in ecstasy, for I have found my True Guru. ||1||[154]

O my mind, remain always with the Lord.
Remain always with the Lord, O my mind, and all sufferings will be forgotten.
He will accept you as His own, and all your affairs will be perfectly arranged.
Our Lord and Master is all-powerful to do all things, so forget Him not.
Says Nanak, O my mind, remain always with the Lord. ||2||

O my True Lord and Master, what is there which is not in Your celestial home?
Everything is in Your home; they receive, unto whom You give.
Constantly singing Your Praises and Glories, Your Name is enshrined in the mind.
The divine melody of the Shabd vibrates for those, within whose minds the Nam abides.
Says Nanak, O my True Lord and Master, what is there which is not in Your home? ||3||
The True Name is my only support.
The True Name is my only support; it satisfies all hunger.
It has brought peace and tranquility to my mind; it has fulfilled all my desires.
I am forever a sacrifice to the Guru, who possesses such glorious greatness.
Says Nanak, listen, O Saints; enshrine love for the Shabd.
The True Name is my only support. ||4||

The Panch (Panj) Shabd, the five primal sounds, vibrate in that blessed house.
In that blessed house, the Shabd vibrates; He infuses His almighty power into it.
Through You, we subdue the five demons of desire, and slay death, the torturer.
Those who have such pre-ordained destiny are attached to the Lord's Name.
Says Nanak, they are at peace, and the unstruck sound current vibrates within their homes. ||5||

Without the true love of devotion, the body is without honor.
The body is dishonored without devotional love; what can the poor wretches do?
No one except You is all-powerful; please bestow Your Mercy, O Lord of all nature.
There is no place of rest, outside the Name; attached to the Shabd, we are embellished with beauty.

Says Nanak, without devotional love, what can the poor wretches do? ||6||
Bliss, bliss - everyone talks of bliss; bliss is known only through the Guru.
Eternal bliss in known only through the Guru, when the Beloved Lord grants His Grace.
Granting His Grace, He pardons our sins; He blesses us with the healing ointment of wisdom.
Those who end attachment from within are adorned with the Shabd, the Word of the True Lord.
Says Nanak, this alone is bliss - bliss which is known through the Guru. ||7||

O Baba, he alone receives it, unto whom You give it.
He alone receives it, unto whom You give it; what can the other poor wretched beings do?
Some are doubtful, wandering in ten directions; some are adorned with attachment to the Nam.
By Guru's Grace, the mind becomes immaculate and pure, for those who follow God's Will.
Says Nanak, he alone receives it, unto whom You give it, O Beloved Lord. ||8||

Come, Beloved Saints, let us speak the Unspoken Speech of the Lord.
How can we speak the Unspoken Speech of the Lord? Through which door will we find Him?
Surrender body, mind, wealth, & everything to the Guru; obey His Order & you will find Him.
Obey the Hukam of the Guru's Command, and sing the True Word of His Bani.
Says Nanak, listen, O Saints, and speak the Unspoken Speech of the Lord. ||9||

O fickle mind, through cleverness, no one has found the Lord.
Through cleverness, no one has found Him; listen, O my mind.
This Maya is so fascinating; because of it, people wander in doubt.
This fascinating Maya was created by the One who has administered this potion.
I am a sacrifice to the One who has made emotional attachment sweet.
Says Nanak, O fickle mind, no one has found Him through cleverness. ||10||

O beloved mind, contemplate the True Lord forever.
This family which you see shall not go along with you.
They shall not go along with you, so why do you focus your attention on them?
Don't do anything that you will regret in the end.
Listen to the Teachings of the True Guru - these shall go along with you.
Says Nanak, O beloved mind, contemplate the True Lord forever. ||11||

O inaccessible and unfathomable Lord, Your limits cannot be found.
No one has found Your limits; only You Yourself know.
All living beings and creatures are Your play; how can anyone describe You?
You speak, and You gaze upon all; You created the Universe.
Says Nanak, You are forever inaccessible; Your limits cannot be found. ||12||

The angelic beings & silent sages search for the Ambrosial Nectar; this is obtained from the Guru.
This Amrit is obtained, when the Guru grants His Grace; He enshrines the Truth within the mind.
All living beings & creatures were created by You; few come to see the Guru & seek His blessing.
Their greed, avarice and egotism are dispelled, and the True Guru seems sweet.
Says Nanak, those with whom the Lord is pleased, obtain the Amrit, through the Guru. ||13||

The lifestyle of the devotees is unique and distinct.
The devotees' lifestyle is unique and distinct; they follow the most difficult path.
They renounce greed, avarice, egotism and desire; they do not talk too much.
The path they take is sharper than a two-edged sword, and finer than a hair.
By Guru's Grace, they shed their selfishness and conceit; their hopes are merged in the Lord.
Says Nanak, the lifestyle of the devotees, in each and every age, is unique and distinct. ||14||

As You make me walk, so do I walk, O my Lord Master; what do I know of Your Glorious Virtues?
As You cause them to walk, they walk - You have placed them on the Path.
In Your Mercy, You attach them to the Nam; they meditate forever on the Lord, Har, Har.
Those whom You cause to listen to Your sermon, find peace in the Gurdwara, the Guru's Gate.
Says Nanak, O my True Lord and Master, you make us walk according to Your Will. ||15||

This song of praise is the Shabd, the most beautiful Word of God.

This beauteous Shabd is the everlasting song of praise, spoken by the True Guru.
This is enshrined in the minds of those who are so pre-destined by the Lord.
Some wander around, babbling on and on, but none obtain Him by babbling.
Says Nanak, the Shabd, this song of praise, has been spoken by the True Guru. ||16||

Those humble beings who meditate on the Lord become pure.
Meditating on the Lord, they become pure; as Gurmukh, they meditate on Him.
They are pure, along with their mothers, fathers, family & friends; their companions are also pure.
Pure are those who speak and those who listen; those who enshrine it within their minds are pure.
Says Nanak, pure and holy are those who, as Gurmukh, meditate on the Lord, Har, Har. ||17||

By religious rituals, intuitive poise is not found; without intuitive poise, skepticism remains.
Skepticism does not depart by contrived actions; everybody is tired of performing these rituals.
The soul is polluted by skepticism; how can it be cleansed?
Wash your mind by attaching it to the Shabd, and keep your consciousness focused on the Lord.
Says Nanak, by Guru's Grace, intuitive poise is produced, and this skepticism is dispelled. ||18||

Inwardly polluted, and outwardly pure.
Those who are outwardly pure and yet polluted within, lose their lives in the gamble.
They contract this terrible disease of desire, and in their minds, they forget about dying.
In the Vedas, the objective is the Naam; but they do not hear this, they wander around like demons.
Says Nanak, those who forsake Truth and cling to falsehood, lose their lives in the gamble. ||19||

Inwardly pure, and outwardly pure.
Those who are outwardly pure and also pure within, through the Guru, perform good deeds.
Not even an iota of falsehood touches them; their hopes are absorbed in the Truth.
Those who earn the jewel of this human life, are the most excellent of merchants.
Says Nanak, those whose minds are pure, abide with the Guru forever. ||20||

If a Sikh turns to the Guru with sincere faith, as sunmukh.
If a Sikh turns to the Guru with sincere faith, as sunmukh, his soul abides with the Guru.
In his heart, he meditates on the lotus feet of the Guru; deep within his soul, he contemplates Him.
Renouncing selfishness & conceit, he remains always to the Guru; he does not know anyone else.
Says Nanak, listen, O Saints: a Sikh turns to the Guru with sincere faith to become sunmukh. ||21||

One who turns away from the True Guru, who becomes baymukh, he shall not find liberation.
He shall not find liberation anywhere else either; go and ask the wise ones about this.
He shall wander through incarnations; without the True Guru, he shall not find liberation.
Liberation is attained, when one is attached to the feet of the True Guru, chanting the Shabd.
Says Nanak, contemplate this and see, that without the True Guru, there is no liberation. ||22||

Come, O beloved Sikhs of the True Guru, and sing the True Word of His Bani.
Sing the Guru's Bani, the supreme Word of Words.
Those who are blessed by the Lord's Glance of Grace - their hearts are imbued with this Bani.
Drink this Nectar, remain in the Lord's Love forever; meditate on the Lord, Sustainer of the world.
Says Nanak, sing this True Bani forever. ||23||

Without the True Guru, other songs are false.
The songs are false without the True Guru; all other songs are false.
The speakers are false, and the listeners are false; those who speak and recite are false.
They continually chant, 'Har, Har' with their tongues, but they do not know what they are saying.
Their consciousness is lured by Maya; they are just reciting mechanically.

Says Nanak, without the True Guru, other songs are false. ||24||

The Word of the Guru's Shabd is a jewel, studded with diamonds.
The mind which is attached to this jewel, merges into the Shabd.
One whose mind is attuned to the Shabd, enshrines love for the True Lord.
He Himself is the diamond, and He Himself is the jewel; one who is blessed, understands its value.
Says Nanak, the Shabd is a jewel, studded with diamonds. ||25||

He Himself created Shiva, Shakti, mind & matter; the Creator subjects them to His Command.
Enforcing His Order, He sees all. How rare are those who, as Gurmukh, come to know Him.
They break their bonds, and attain liberation; they enshrine the Shabd within their minds.
Those whom the Lord makes Gurmukh, lovingly focus their consciousness on the One Lord.
Says Nanak, He Himself is the Creator; He Himself reveals the Hukam of His Command. ||26||
The Simritees & Shastras discriminate between good & evil, but don't know the essence of reality.
They do not know the true essence of reality without the Guru; they do not know the true essence.
The world is asleep in the three modes and doubt; it passes the night of its life sleeping.
The humble remain aware, within whose minds, the Lord abides; they chant the Guru's Bani.
Says Nanak, they alone obtain the essence of reality, who night and day remain lovingly absorbed in the Lord; they pass the night of their life awake and aware. ||27||

He nourished us in the mother's womb; why erase Him from the mind?
Why forget such a Great Giver, who gave us sustenance in the fire of the womb?
Nothing can harm one, whom the Lord inspires to embrace His Love.
He Himself is the love, and He Himself is the embrace; the Gurmukh contemplates Him forever.
Says Nanak, why forget such a Great Giver from the mind? ||28||

As is the fire within the womb, so is Maya outside.
The fire of Maya is one and the same; the Creator has staged this play.
According to His Will, the child is born, and the family is very pleased.
Love for the Lord wears off & the child becomes attached to desires; Maya's script runs its course.
This is Maya, by which the Lord is forgotten; emotional attachment and love of duality well up.
Says Nanak, by Guru's Grace, those who enshrine love for the Lord find Him, amidst Maya. ||29||

The Lord Himself is priceless; His worth cannot be estimated.
His worth cannot be estimated, even though people have grown weary of trying.
If you meet such a True Guru, offer your head to Him; your selfishness & conceit will be ended.
Your soul belongs to Him; remain united with Him, and the Lord will come to dwell in your mind.
The Lord Himself is priceless; very fortunate are those, O Nanak, who attain to the Lord. ||30||

The Lord is my capital; my mind is the merchant.
The Lord is my capital, and my mind is the merchant; through the True Guru, I know my capital.
Meditate continually on the Lord, Har, Har, O my soul, and you shall collect your profits daily.
This wealth is obtained by those who are pleasing to the Lord's Will.
Says Nanak, the Lord is my capital, and my mind is the merchant. ||31||

O my tongue, you are engrossed in other tastes, but your thirsty desire is not quenched.
Your thirst shall not be quenched by any means, until you attain the subtle essence of the Lord.
If you obtain the essence of the Lord, drink it in, you shall not be troubled by desire again.
This subtle essence of the Lord is obtained by good karma, when one comes to meet the True Guru.
Says Nanak, all other tastes are forgotten, when the Lord comes to dwell within the mind. ||32||

O my body, the Lord infused His Light into you, and then you came into the world.

The Lord infused His Light into you, and then you came into the world.
The Lord Himself is your mother and father; He created beings and revealed the world to them.
By Guru's Grace, some understand, and then it's a show; it seems like just a show.
Says Nanak, He laid foundations of the Universe, infused His Light & you entered the world. ||33||

O my mind has become joyful, hearing of God's coming.
Sing songs of joy to welcome the Lord, O my companions; my household is the Lord's Mansion.
Sing the songs of joy & welcome the Lord, my companions; sorrow & suffering will not afflict you.
Blessed is that day, when I am attached to the Guru's feet and meditate on my Husband Lord.
I now know the unstruck sound & Word of the Shabad; I enjoy the Lord's sublime essence.
Says Nanak, God Himself has met me; He is the Doer, the Cause of causes. ||34||

O my body, why have you come into this world? What actions have you committed?
And what actions have you committed, O my body, since you came into this world?
The Lord who formed your form - you have not enshrined that Lord in your mind.
By Guru's Grace, the Lord abides within the mind, and one's pre-ordained destiny is fulfilled.
Says Nanak, this body is adorned when consciousness is focused on the True Guru. ||35||

O my eyes, the Lord has infused His Light into you; do not look upon any other than the Lord.
Do not look upon any other than the Lord; the Lord alone is worthy of beholding.
This whole world which you see is the image of the Lord; only the image of the Lord is seen.
By Guru's Grace, I understand and I see only the One Lord; there is no one except the Lord.
Says Nanak, these eyes were blind; but meeting the True Guru, they became all-seeing. ||36||

O my ears, you were created only to hear the Truth.
To hear the Truth, you were created and attached to the body; listen to the True Bani.
Hearing it, the mind and body are rejuvenated and the tongue is absorbed in Ambrosial Nectar.
The True Lord is unseen and wondrous; His state cannot be described.
Says Nanak, listen to the Ambrosial Nam, become holy; you were created only to hear Truth. ||37||

The Lord placed the soul in cave of the body & blew the breath of life into that musical instrument.
He blew breath of life into the body revealing nine doors; He kept the Tenth Door hidden.
Through the Guru's Gate, some are blessed with loving faith & the Tenth Door is revealed to them.
There are many images of the Lord, and the nine treasures of the Nam; His limits cannot be found.
Says Nanak, the Lord placed the soul in the body & blew the breath of life into the body. ||38||

Sing this true song of praise in the true home of your soul.
Sing the song of praise in your true home; meditate there on the True Lord forever.
They meditate on You, O True Lord, those pleasing to Your Will; as Gurmukh, they understand.
This Truth is the Lord and Master of all; whoever is blessed, obtains it.
Says Nanak, sing the true song of praise in the true home of your soul. ||39||

Listen to the song of bliss, O most fortunate ones; all your longings shall be fulfilled.
I have obtained the Supreme Lord God, and all sorrows have been forgotten.
Pain, illness and suffering have departed, listening to the True Bani.
The Saints and their friends are in ecstasy, knowing the Perfect Guru.
Pure are the listeners, and pure are the speakers; the True Guru is all-pervading and permeating.
Prays Nanak, touching the Guru's Feet, the unstruck sound current of the celestial bugles vibrates and resounds. ||40||1||[155]

REHIRAS SAHIB

Contained within this evening prayer are the contributions of 5 different Gurus: *Guru Nanak, Guru Amardas, Guru Ram Das, Guru Arjun Dev* and *Guru Gobind Singh*. Traditionally, this bani is recited with the family together, after each has returned home from a days work. It is a way of giving thanks to God for another successful day.[156]

Rehiras

Slok Mehla Pehila (1)

Dūk daru sūk rog bheya ja sūk tam no hoy
Tūn karta karma mey nahi ja hau kari na hoy ||1||
Balihari kudrat vasi-e tera ant na jey lakia ||1|| Rahao

Jat mey jot jot mey jata akal kala barpur rehia
Tūn sacha sahïb sifat sualio jïn kïti so par peya
Kahu Nanïk karte kia bata
jo kïch karma sūkar rehia ||2||

Sodar Rag Asa Mehla Pehila (1)

Do dar teyra keyha so gar keyha jït bhai sarab samaley
Vajey tey-rey nad aneyk asanka key-tey tey-rey vavïn-harey
Keytey tey-rey rag pari sio kahi-ahi key-tey tey-rey gavan-harey
Gavan tūd-no pavan pani bey-santar gavey raja daram du-arey
Gavan tūd-no chït gūpat lïk janan lïk lïk daram bicharey
Gavan tūd-no isar barma deyvi sohan tey-rey sada savarey
Gavan tūd-no ïndr ïndrasan bey-tey deyv tia dar naley
Gavan tūd-no sïd samadi andar gavan tūd-no sad bicharey
Gavan tūd-no jati sati santoki gavan tūd-no vir kara-rey
Gavan tūd-no pandit paran raki-sur jūg jūg veyda naley
Gavan tūd-no mohani-a man mohan surga mach pi-a-ley
Gavan tūd-no ratan upa-ey tey-rey atsat tirat naley
Gaveh tūd-no jod mahabal sūra gavey tūd-no kani charey
Gaveh tūd-no kand mandal varbanda kar kar rakey tere darey
Sey tūd-no gaveh jo-tūd bavan ratey tey-rey bagat rasaley
Hor key-tey gavan sey mey chït na avan Nanïk ki-a bicharey
So-i so-i sada sach sahïb sacha sachi nai
Hey bi hosi jai na jasi rachna jïn racha-i
Rangi rangi bati kar kar jïnsi mai-a jïn ūpa-i
Kar kar dey-key kita apna jïv tïs di vadia-i
Jo tïs bavey so-i karsi fir hūkam na karna jai
So patïsa saha patïsa-ïb Nanïk rahan rajai ||1||

Asa Mehla Pehila (1)

114

Sūn vada akey sab koi key-vad vada dita ho-i
Kimat pa-ey na kahia jai
Keh-ney valey tey-rey rahey sama-i ||1||
Vadey mey-rey sahïb-a gahir gambira gūni gahira
Ko-ey na janey teyra keyta keyvad chira ||1|| Rahao

Sab surti mil surat kama-i
Sab kimat mil kimat pai
Gi-ani di-ani gur gura-i
Kehen na jai teyri tïl vadia-i ||2||

Sab sat sab tap sab changa-ia
Sïda purk-ha kia vadia-ia
Tūd vïn sïdi kïney na pa-ia
Karm mïley nahi tak raha-ia ||3||

Akan vala kia veychara
Sïfti barey tey-rey bandara
Jïs tu de tïsey kia chara
Nanïk sach savaran-hara ||4||2||

Asa Mehla Pehila (1)

Aka jiva vïsrey mar ja-o
Akan a-uka sacha na-o
Sachey nam ki lagey būk
Ut būkey ka-ey chali-ai dūk ||1||
So kio vïsrey meyri ma-i
Sacha sahïb sachey na-i ||1|| Rahao
Sachey nam ki tïl vadia-i
Aak takey kimat nahi pa-i
Jey sab mïl key akan pa-i
Vada na hovey gat na ja-i ||2||

Na-o marey na hovey sog
Deyda rehe na chūkey bog
Gūn ey-ho hor nahi ko-i
Na ko hoa na ko ho-i ||3||

Jeyvad aap teyvad teyri dat
Jïn dïn kar key ki-ti rat
Kasam vïsarey tey kamjat
Nanïk navey baj sanat ||4||3||

Rag Gūjri Mehla Chauta (4)

Har key jan Satïgur sat pūrka
Bïna-o kara-o gur pas

115

Ham kirey kirm Satïgur sarna-i
Kar da-ia nam pargas ||1||
Mey-rey mit Gurdeyv
Mo ka-o ram nam pargas
Gurmat nam meyra parn saka-i
Har kirït hamri rehiras ||1|| Rahao

Har jan key vad bag vadey-rey
Jïn har har sarda har pi-as
Har har nam mïley trïp-tasahi
Mïl sangat gūn pargas ||2||

Jïn har har har ras nam
Na pai-a tey bha-gin jam pas
Jo Satïgur saran sangat nahi
A-ey darïg jivey darïg jivas ||3||

Jïn har jan Satïgur sangat
Pa-i tïn dur mastïk lïkia lïkas
Dhan Dhan Sat-sangat jït har ras
Pai-a mïl jan Nanïk nam pargas ||4||4||

Rag Gūjri Mehla Panjva (5)

Kahey rey man chït-vehi
Udam ja a-har har jio pari-a
Sel patar me jant upa-ey
Ta ka rïjak agey kar dari-a ||1||
Meyrey mad-hao ji sat-sangat mïley so tari-a
Gur prasad parm pad pai-a sūkey kasat haria ||1|| Rahao

Janan pïta lok sūt banita
Koi na kïs ki dhari-a
Sïr sïr rïjak samba-hey
Takur kahey man bao kari-a ||2||

Udey ūd avey sey kosa tïs
Pachey bach-rey chari-a
Tïn kavan kalavey kavan chūgavey
Man me sïmran kari-a ||3||

Sab nïdan das-asat sïdan
Takur kar tal dari-a
Jan Nanïk bal bal sad bal jai-ey
Teyra ant na paravari-a ||4||5||

Rag Asa Mehla Chauta So Purkh

Ek ong kar Satïgur prasad
So Purk niranjan har purk

116

Niranjan har agma agam apara
Sab di-ave sab di-ave
Tūd ji har sachey sirjan-hara
Sab ji-a tūmarey ji tu ji-a ka datara
Har di-avahu santahu ji sab dūk visaran-hara ||1||
Har apey takur har apey
Seyvek ji ki-a Nanïk jant vichara
Tu gat gat antar sarab
Nirantar ji har eyko purk samana
Ek datey-ek bey-kari ji
Sab teyrey choj vidana
Tu apey data apey bhūgta ji ha-o
Tūd bïn avar na jana
Tu par-brahm bey-ant bey-ant ji
Teyrey ki-a gūn-ak vakana
Jo sey-veh jo sey-veh
Tūd ji jan Nanïk tïn kūrbana ||2||

Har di-avahe har di-avahe
Tūd ji sey jan jūg meh sūkvasi

Sey mūkat sey mūkat ba-ey jïn
Har dia-ia ji tïn tūti jïm ki fasi
Jïn nirbao jïn har nirbao dia-ia ji
Tïn ka ba-o sab gavasi
Jïn seyvi-a jïn seyvi-a meyra
Har ji tey har har rūp samasi
Sey dan sey dan jïn har dia-ia ji
Jan Nanïk tïn bal jasi ||3||

Teyri bagat teyri bagat bandar ji
Barey bi-ant bey-anta
Teyrey bagat teyrey bagat salahan tūd ji
Har anek aneyk ananta
Teyri anek teyri anek karahi har pūja ji
Tap tapeh japeh Bey-anta
Teyrey anek teyrey anek pareh baho sïmrat sasat ji
Kar kïri-a kat karam karanta
Sey bagat sey bagat baley jan Nanïk Ji
Jo baveh meyrey har bagvanta ||4||

Tu aad purk aprampar karta ji
Tūd jeyvad avar na ko-i
Tu jūg jūg eyko sada sada tu eyko ji
Tu nehechal karta so-i
Tūd apey bavey so-i vartey ji
Tu apey karahi so ho-i

117

Tūd apey srïst sab ūpa-i ji
Tūd apey siraj sab go-i
Jan Nanïk gūn gavey kartey key ji
Jo sab-sey ka jano-i ||5||1||

Asa Mehla Chauta (4)

Tūn karta sachiar meyda sa-i
Jo ta-o bavey so-i tisi jo tu-de so-i hao pa-i ||1|| Rahao

Sab teyri tu sabni dia-ia
Jïs no kirpa kare-hi tïn nam ratan pai-a
Gurmūk lada man-mūk gavai-a
Tūd aap vichori-a aap mïlai-a ||1||

Tu dari-ao sab tūj hi mahi
Tūj bïn dūja ko-i nahi
Jia jant sab teyra khel
Vijog mïl vichuri-a sanjogi mel ||2||

Jïs no tu jana-eh so-i jan janey
Har gūn sad hi aak vakaney
Jïn har seyvi-a tïn sūk pai-a
Sahajey hi har nam samai-a ||3||

Tu apey karta teyra kia sab ho-i
Tūd bïn dūja avar na ko-i
Tu kar kar vey-key jana-hi so-i
Jan Nanïk gurmūk pargat ho-i ||4||2||

Asa Mehla pehila (1)

Tït saravrar-he ba-iley nivasa pani pavïk tïney kia
Pankaj mopag nahi chaley ham deyka ta dūbi-aley ||1||
Man eyk na cheytas mūr mana
Har bïsrat tey-rey gūn gali-a ||1|| Rahao

Na ha-o jati sati nahi parhi-a
Mūrk mūgda janam bai-a
Pranavat Nanïk tïn ki sarna jïn tu nahi vïsari-a ||2||3||

Asa Mehla Panjva (5)

Ba-i parapat manūk dey-huri-a
Gobïnd mïlan ki-eh teyri bai-a
Avar kaj tey-rey kïtey na kam
Mïl sad-sangat bhaj key-val nam ||1||
Saran-jam lag bhav-jal taran key

118

Janam bari-ta jat rang mai-a key ||1|| Rahao

Jap tap sanjam daram na kamai-a
Seyva sad na jani-a har rai-a
Keho Nanïk ham nich karama
Saran parey ki rako sarma ||2||4||

Patïsahi Dasvi (10)

Hamari karo hat dey racha
Pūrn ho-i chït ki icha
Tav charanan man rehe hamara
Apana jan karo pratipara ||1||

Hamarey dūsht sabey tūm gava-ho
Aap hat dey mohi bachava-ho
Sūki basey moro mari-vara
Seyvak sïk-ya sabey karatara ||2||

Mo racha nïj kar dey kari-ey
Sab bey-ran ko aj san-gari-ey
Pūrn ho-i hamari asa
Tor bajan ki rehe pi-asa ||3||

Tūma-hi chas ko-i avar na dia-u
Jo bar cha-ho tūm tey pa-u
Sey-val sïk-ya hamarey tari-ai
Chūn chūn satr hamarey mari-ai ||4||

Aap hat di mūjey ūbari-ey
Marn kal ka tras nivari-ey
Hūjo sada hamarey pacha
Sri asi-dūj ju kari-yaho racha ||5||

Rak leyo muhi rakan-harey
Sahïb sant sahai piya-rey
Din bandu dūshtan key hanta
Tūma-ho pure chatr das kanta ||6||

Kal pai brah-ma būd dara
Kal pai shiva-ju avatara
Kal pai kar bisan prakasa
Sakal kal ka kia tamasa ||7||

Javan kal jogi sïv ki-o
Bey-draj brah-ma ju ti-o
Javan kal sab lok savara

119

Namaskar hey ta-hi hamara ||8||

Javan kal sab jagat bani-yo
Deyv deyt ja-chan ūpa-jeyo
Aad ant ey-key avatara
So-i guru sama-ji ya-ho hamara ||9||

Namaskar tïs hi ko hamari
Sakal praja jïn aap savari
Sïv-akan ko siv-agūn sūk di-o
Satran ko pal mo bad ki-o ||10||

Gat Gat key antar ki janat
Bha-ley burey ki pir pachanat
Chi-ti tey kūnchar astūla
Sab par kirpa drïsht kar fūla ||11||

Santan dūk pa-ey tey dūki
Sūk pa-ey sadan key sūki
Eyk eyk ki pir pachan-ey
Gat gat key pat pat ki janey ||12||

Jab ūdaka-rak kara kara-tara
Praja dart tab deyj apara
Jab akar-ak kart ho kaba-hu
Tūm mey mïlat dey dar saba-hu ||13||

Jey-tey badan sri-sat sab darey
Aap aap-ni būj ūcharey
Tūm saba-hi tey rehet niralam
Janat beyd beyd ar alam ||14||

Nirankar nri-bikar nir-alam
Aad anil anad asanb
Ta ka mura ūcha-rat beyda
Ja kau beyv pavat beyda ||15||

Ta kau kar pahen anu-manït
Maha mura kach beyd na janat
Maha-deyv kau kehet sada shïv
Nirankar ka chi-nat nahi bïv ||16||

Aap aap-ni būd hey jeyti
Baranat bïn bïn tu-hi teyti
Tūmara laka na jai pasara
Ke bïd saja pratam sansara ||17||

Ey-key rūp anūp sarūpa
Rank beyo rav kehe būpa
Andaj jey-raj sey-taj ki-ni
Uta-baj kehen bahur rach di-ni ||18||

Kahu fūl raja havey beyta
Kahu sïmat biyo sankar i-key-ta
Sagari srïst dïka-i achan-bav
Aad jūgad sarūp su-yan-bav ||19||

Aab racha meyri tūm karo
Sïk ubar asïk sang-haro
Dūsht jitey utavat uta-pata
Sakal maleych karo ran gata ||20||

Jey asi-dūj tav sarni parey
Tïn key dūsht dūkat havey marey
Purk javan pag parey ti-harey
Tïn key tūm sankat sab tarey ||21||

Jo kal ko ek bar di-ey hey
Ta key kal nikat na-hi ey-hey
Racha ho-i ta-hi sab kala
Dūsht arïsht tarey tata-kala ||22||

Kirpa drïsht tan ja-hi ni-hari-ho
Ta key tap tanïk mo hari-ho
Rïd sïd gar mo sab jo-i
Dūsht cha chavey sakey na ko-i ||23||

Eyk bar jïn tūmey san-bhara
Kal fas tey ta-hi u-bara
Jïn nar nam ti-haro kahae
Darïd dūsht dok tey rahae ||24||

Kar-hag keyt mey saran ti-hari
Aap hat dey ley-ho u-bari
Sarab ta-ur mo hoho saha-i
Dūsht dok tey ley bacha-i ||25||

Svaye

Pane ge-hae jab tae tūma-rae tab tae
Ku-ank tarey ne-hi aneyo
Ram rehem puran kuran anek
Kehen mat eyk na mana-yo
Sïmrït shastr beyd sabey bao
Beyd kahey ham eyk na ja-neyo

121

Sri asapan kripa tūmari kar
Mey na ke-heyo sab to-hi bak-haneyo

Doh-ra

Sagal duar ka-o chad key gai-o tu-haro duar
Bani gahey ki laj as Gobïnd das tuhar

Ramkali Mehla Tija (3) Anand

Ek ong kar Satïgur prasad

Anand bai-a meyri mai Satïguru mey pai-a
Satïgur ta pa-ia sahej seyti man vaji-a vadha-ia
Rag ratan parvar pari-a shabd gavana-ia
Shabdo ta gavaho Hari keyra man jïnee vasa-ia
Kahey Nanïk anand hoa Satïguru mey pa-ia ||1||

Ay man meyri-a tu sada rahu har naley
Har nal rahu tu man mey-rey dūkh sab visarna
Angikar oh karey teyra karaj sab savarna
Sabna gala samrat su-ami so ki-o manhu visarey
Kahey Nanïk man mey-rey sada rahu har naley ||2||

Sachey sahiba kia nahi gar tey-rey
Gar ta tey-rey sab kïch hey jïs deh so pavey
Sada sïfat sala teyri nam man vasava-ey
Nam jïn key man vasia vajey sabd ganey-rey
Kahey Nanïk sachey sahïb kia nahi gar tey-rey ||3||

Sacha nam meyra adharo
Sach nam adhar meyra jïn bhūka sab gava-ia
Kar sat sūk mana-ey vasi-a jïn icha sab puja-ia
Sada kurban kita Guru vitahau jïs dia-eyhi vadia-ia
Kahey Nanïk sūnu santahu sabd darahu pi-aro
Sacha Nam meyra adharo ||4||
Vajey panch sabd tït gar sabagey
Gar sabagey sabd vajey kala jït gar daria
Panch dūt tūd vas kitey kal kantak maria
Dhur karam pa-ia tūd jïn ka-o se nam har key lagey
Kahey Nanïk ta sūk hoa tït gar anad vajey ||5||

Anad sūnū vad-bagio sagal manorat pūrey
Parbarm parab pa-ia ūtrey sagal visūrey
Dūk rog santap ūtrey sūni sachi bani
Sant sajan ba-ey sarsey pūrey Gur tey jani
Sūntey pūnit katey pavït Satïgur rahia barpurey
Bïnvant Nanïk Gur charn lagey vajey anad tūrey ||40||1||

122

Mūndavani Mehla Panjva (5)

Tal vïch tïn vastu pai-o sat santok vicharo
Amrït nam takur ka pai-o jïs ka sabas ad-haro
Jey ko kavey jey ko būnch-ey tïs ka ho-ey ud-haro
Ey vasït taji na jai nït nït rak ur dharo
Tam sansar charn lag tari-ey
Sab Nanïk brahm pasaro ||1||

Slok Mehla Panjava (5)

Teyra kita jato nahi meyno jog kito-i
Mey nir-guni arey ko gūn nahi apey taras pai-o-i
Taras pai-a mi-haramat ho-i Satïgur sajan mïli-a
Nanïk nam mïley tan jiva tan man tïvey hari-a ||1||

Pauri Mehla Panjva (5)

Tïtey tu samrat jïtey ko-e na-hi
O-tey teri rak agni ūdar ma-hi
Sūn key jam ke dūt ne terey chadi ja-hi
Baujal bikam asga gur sabdi par pa-hi
Jïn kau lagi pias amrït se-e ka-hi
Kal mey e-ho pūn gūn Govïnd ga-hi
Sab-sey no kirpal samaley sa-hi sa-hi
Birta ko-e na ja-e je avey tūd a-hi ||9||

Slok Mehla Panjva (5)

Antar gur ara-dana jiva jap gur na-o
Netri Satïgur pek-na sravani su-nana gur na-o
Satïgur seti ratia darga paley ta-o
Kahu Nanïk kirpa karey jïs no-eh vat de-e
Jag mey ūtam kad-hey vir-ley key ke-e ||1||

Mehla Panjva (5)

Rak-e Rakana-har Aap Ubarian
Gur Ki Peri Pai-e Kaj Savarian
Ho-a Aap Dai-al Manaho Na Vïsarian
Sad Jana Ke Sang Bavajal Tarian
Sakat Nïndak Dusht Kïn Ma-e Bïdarian
Tïs Sahïb Ki Teyk Nanïk Mane Ma-e
Jïs Sïmrat Sūk O-e Sagaley Dūk Ja-e ||2||

Rehiras
Sermon from the First Guru

Pain is the medicine, material joy is the disease; when there are worldly pleasures, there is not love for God. You are the Creator, I am nothing; If I attempt to do something, nothing comes out of it. ||1||
I am a sacrifice to You. You reside in nature in Your Omnipotence; Your end cannot be seen. ||1|| Pause *(The purpose of each Rahao, or Pause, is to allow a moment to contemplate what has just been read)*

Your light pervades the creation and the creation is contained in Your light. Your own Supreme Power fills the inanimate and animate creation. You are the True Lord, Your praise is most beautiful; whosoever utters Your praise crosses the world ocean. Nanak utters words of praise of the Creator. Whatever is to be done by God will be done. ||2||

One Universal Creator God. By The Grace Of The True Guru:

Where is That Door of Yours, and where is That Home, in which You sit and take care of all? The Sound-Current of the Nad vibrates there for You, and countless musicians play all sorts of instruments there for You. There are so many Ragas and musical harmonies to You; so many minstrels sing hymns of You. Wind, water and fire sing of You. The Righteous Judge of Dharma sings at Your Door. Chitr and Gupat, the angels of the conscious and the subconscious who keep the record of actions, and the Righteous Judge of Dharma who reads this record, sing of You. Shiva, Brahma and the Goddess of Beauty, ever adorned by You, sing of You. Indra, seated on His Throne, sings of You, with the deities at Your Door. The Siddhas in Samadhi sing of You; the Sadhus sing of You in contemplation. The celibates, the fanatics, and the peacefully accepting sing of You; the fearless warriors sing of You. The Pandits, the religious scholars who recite the Vedas, with the supreme sages of all the ages, sing of You. The Mohinis, the enchanting heavenly beauties who entice hearts in paradise, in this world, and in the underworld of the subconscious, sing of You. The celestial jewels created by You, and the sixty-eight sacred shrines of pilgrimage, sing of You. The brave and mighty warriors sing of You. The spiritual heroes and the four sources of creation sing of You. The worlds, solar systems and galaxies, created and arranged by Your Hand, sing of You. They alone sing of You, who are pleasing to Your Will. Your devotees are imbued with Your Sublime Essence. So many others sing of You, they do not come to mind. O Nanak, how can I think of them all? That True Lord is True, forever True, and True is His Name. He is, and shall always be. He shall not depart, even when this Universe which He has created departs. He created the world, with its various colors, species of beings, and the variety of Maya. Having created the creation, He watches over it Himself, by His Greatness. He does whatever He pleases. No one can issue any order to Him. He is the King, the King of kings, the Supreme Lord and Master of kings. Nanak remains subject to His Will. ||1||

Asa, from the First Guru *(These denote which Rag, or musical melodic structure, is to be applied to the following stanza & from which Guru this hymn comes)*

Hearing of His Greatness, everyone calls Him Great. But just how Great His Greatness is; this is known only to those who have seen Him. His Value cannot be estimated; He cannot be described. Those who describe You, Lord, remain immersed and absorbed in You.||1||
O my Great Lord and Master of Unfathomable Depth, You are the Ocean of Excellence. No one knows the extent or the vastness of Your Expanse. ||1||Pause||

All the intuitives met and practiced intuitive meditation. All the appraisers met and made the appraisal. The spiritual teachers, the teachers of meditation, and the teachers of teachers - they cannot describe even an iota of Your Greatness. ||2||

All Truth, all austere discipline, all goodness, all the great, miraculous, spiritual powers of the Siddhas; without You, no one has attained such powers. They are received only by Your Grace. No one can block them or stop their flow. ||3||

What can the poor helpless creatures do? Your Praises are overflowing with Your Treasures. Those, unto whom You give; how can they think of any other? O Nanak, the True One embellishes and exalts. ||4||2||

Asa, from the First Guru

Chanting it, I live; forgetting it, I die. It is so difficult to chant the True Name. If someone feels hunger for the True Name, that hunger shall consume his pain. ||1||
How can I forget Him, O my mother? True is the Master, True is His Name. ||1||Pause||

Trying to describe even an iota of the Greatness of the True Name, people have grown weary, but they have not been able to evaluate it. Even if everyone were to gather together and speak of Him, He would not become any greater or any lesser. ||2||

That Lord does not die; there is no reason to mourn. He continues to give, and His Provisions never run short. This Virtue is His alone; there is no other like Him. There never has been, and there never will be. ||3||

As Great as You are, O Lord, so Great are Your Gifts. The One who created the day also created the night. Those who forget their Lord and Master are vile and despicable. O Nanak, without the Name, they are wretched outcasts. ||4||3||

Gujri, from the Fourth Guru

O humble servant of the Lord, O True Guru, O True Primal Being: I offer my humble prayer to You, O Guru. I am a mere insect, a worm. O True Guru, I seek Your Sanctuary. Please be merciful, and bless me with the Light of the Nam, the Name of the Lord. ||1||
O my Best Friend, O Divine Guru, please enlighten me with the Name of the Lord. Through the Guru's Teachings, the Nam is my breath of life. The Kirtan of the Lord's Praise is my life's occupation. ||1||Pause||

The servants of the Lord have the greatest good fortune; they have faith in the Lord, and a longing for the Lord. Obtaining the Name of the Lord, Har, Har, they are satisfied; joining the Sangat, the Blessed Congregation, their virtues shine forth. ||2||

Those who have not obtained the Sublime Essence of the Name of the Lord, Har, Har, Har, are most unfortunate; they are led away by the Messenger of Death. Those who have not sought the Sanctuary of the True Guru and the Sangat, the Holy Congregation, cursed are their lives, and cursed are their hopes of life. ||3||

Those humble servants of the Lord who have attained the Company of the True Guru, have such pre-ordained destiny inscribed on their foreheads. Blessed, blessed is the Sat Sangat, the True Congregation, where the Lord's Essence is obtained. Meeting with His humble servant, O Nanak, the Light of the Nam shines forth. ||4||4||

Gujri, from the Fifth Guru

Why, O mind, do you plot and plan, when the Dear Lord Himself provides for your care? From rocks and stones He created living beings; He places their nourishment before them. ||1||

125

O my Dear Lord of souls, one who joins the Sat Sangat, the True Congregation, is saved. By Guru's Grace, the supreme status is obtained, and the dry wood blossoms forth again in lush greenery. ||1||Pause||

Mothers, fathers, friends, children and spouses; no one is the support of anyone else. For each and every person, our Lord and Master provides sustenance. Why are you so afraid, O mind? ||2||

The flamingoes fly hundreds of miles, leaving their young ones behind. Who feeds them, and who teaches them to feed themselves? Have you ever thought of this in your mind? ||3||
All the nine treasures and the eighteen supernatural powers are held by our Lord and Master in the Palm of His Hand. Servant Nanak is devoted, dedicated, forever a sacrifice to You, Lord. Your Expanse has no limit, no boundary. ||4||5||

Asa, from the Fourth Guru, So Purk ~ That Primal Being

One Universal Creator God; By The Grace Of The True Guru

That Primal Being is Immaculate and Pure. The Lord, the Primal Being, is Immaculate and Pure. The Lord is Inaccessible, Unreachable and Unrivalled. All meditate; all meditate on You, Dear Lord, O True Creator Lord. All living beings are Yours; You are the Giver of all souls. Meditate on the Lord, O Saints; He is the Dispeller of all sorrow. The Lord Himself is the Master, the Lord Himself is the Servant. O Nanak, the poor beings are wretched and miserable! ||1||

You are constant in each and every heart, and in all things. O Dear Lord, you are the One. Some are givers, and some are beggars. This is all Your Wondrous Play. You Yourself are the Giver, and You Yourself are the Enjoyer. I know no other than You. You are the Supreme Lord God, Limitless and Infinite. What Virtues of Yours can I speak of and describe? Unto those who serve You, Dear Lord, servant Nanak is a sacrifice. ||2||

Those who meditate on You, Lord; Those who meditate on You, Those humble beings dwell in peace in this world. They are liberated; They are liberated those, those who meditate on the Lord. For them, the noose of death is cut away. Those who meditate on the Fearless One, on the Fearless Lord, all their fears are dispelled. Those who serve; Those who serve my Dear Lord, are absorbed into the Being of the Lord, Har, Har. Blessed are they; blessed are they, who meditate on their Dear Lord. Servant Nanak is a sacrifice to them. ||3||

Devotion to You; Devotion to You, is a treasure overflowing, infinite and beyond measure. Your devotees; Your devotees praise You, Dear Lord, in many and countless ways. For You, many; for You, so very many perform worship services, O Dear Infinite Lord; they practice disciplined meditation and chant endlessly. For You, many; For You, so very many read the various Simritees and Shastras. They perform rituals and religious rites. Those devotees; Those devotees are sublime, O servant Nanak, who are pleasing to my Dear Lord God. ||4||

You are the Primal Being, the Most Wonderful Creator. There is no other as Great as You. Age after age, You are the One. Forever and ever, You are the One. You never change, O Creator Lord. Everything happens according to Your Will. You accomplish all that occurs. You created the entire universe, and having fashioned it, You, Yourself, shall destroy it all. Servant Nanak sings the Glorious Praises of the Dear Creator, the Knower of all. ||5||1||

Asa, from the Fourth Guru

You are the True Creator, my Lord and Master

Whatever pleases You comes to pass. As You give, so do we receive. ||1||Pause||
All belong to You, all meditate on you. Those who are blessed with Your Mercy obtain the Jewel of the Nam, the Name of the Lord. The Gurmukhs obtain it, and the self-willed manmukhs lose it. You separate them from Yourself, and You Yourself reunite with them again. ||1||

You are the River of Life; all are within You. There is no one except You. All living beings are Your playthings. The separated ones meet, and by great good fortune, those suffering in separation are reunited once again. ||2||

They alone understand, whom You inspire to understand; They continually chant and repeat the Lord's Praises. Those who serve You find peace. They are intuitively absorbed into the Lord's Name. ||3||

You are the Creator. Everything that happens is by Your Doing. There is no one except You. You created the creation; You behold it and understand it. O servant Nanak, the Lord is revealed through the Gurmukh, the Living Expression of the Guru's Word. ||4||2||

Asa, from the First Guru

In that pool, people have made their homes, but the water there is as hot as fire! In the swamp of emotional attachment, their feet cannot move. I have seen them drowning there. ||1||

In your mind, you do not remember the One Lord-you fool! You have forgotten the Lord; Your virtues shall wither away. ||1||Pause||

I am not celibate, nor truthful, nor scholarly. I was born foolish and ignorant into this world. Prays Nanak, I seek the Sanctuary of those who have not forgotten You, O Lord! ||2||3||

Asa, from the Fifth Guru

This human body has been given to you. This is your chance to meet the Lord of the Universe. Nothing else will work. Join the Sat Sangat, the Company of the Holy; Vibrate and meditate on the Jewel of the Nam. ||1||
Make every effort to cross over this terrifying world-ocean. You are squandering this life uselessly in the love of Maya. ||1||Pause||

I have not practiced meditation, self-discipline, self-restraint or righteous living. I have not served the Holy; I have not acknowledged the Lord, my King. Says Nanak, my actions are contemptible! O Lord, I seek Your Sanctuary; please, preserve my honor! ||2||4||

Hymn from The Tenth Guru

Kabyo Bach Beyanti Chaupai (to be read like a poem)

Please give me Your Hand, Lord, and protect me
Please fulfill my mind's desires
Let my mind remain attached to Your Lotus Feet
Please make me Your Own, and cherish me ||1||
Please destroy all my enemies
Give me Your Hand, and save me
May my family live in peace
May all my serviceful Sikhs dwell in peace, O Creator Lord ||2||

Protect me with Your All-Powerful Arm
May all my enemies be destroyed today
May my hopes be fulfilled
May my thirst for chanting Your Name continue ||3||

May I never forsake You, May I meditate only on You
May I obtain from You the gifts I wish for
Help my serviceful Sikhs cross over
Single out my enemies and kill them ||4||

Please, give me Your Hand and save me
Destroy the fear of death from within
Please be always on my side
O Wielder of the Great Sword of Justice, please protect me; Protect me, O Protector Lord ||5||

O Beloved Lord and Master, Helper and Support of the Saints
O Friend of the poor, Destroyer of tyrants
You are the Lord of the fourteen worlds ||6||

As ordained by God, Brahma obtained a body
As ordained by God, Shiva became incarnate
As ordained by God, Vishnu appeared
All this is the Play of God ||7||

God created the Yogi Shiva
He created Brahma, the king of the Vedas
He fashioned the whole world
I bow in humble adoration to Him ||8||

God created the whole world
He created the demi-gods, demons and spirits
From beginning to end, He is the One Incarnate
Let everyone know, that He is my Guru ||9||

I humbly bow to Him
He Himself has created all beings
He bestows happiness on His virtuous servants
He destroys the evil and the wicked in an instant ||10||

He knows what is within each and every heart
He knows the sufferings of the good and the bad
From the tiny ant, to the huge elephant
Upon all, He casts His Glance of Grace ||11||

When His Saints endure suffering, He suffers
When the Holy are happy, He is happy
He knows the cares of each and every one
He knows each and every secret of each and every heart ||12||

When the Creator projects His Creative Power
His Creation is created in countless forms
And when He draws His Creation into Himself again

All living beings are re-absorbed into Him ||13||

All beings who have come into the world
Describe God according to their own understanding
O Lord, You remain detached from everything
Only the learned and the wise understand this ||14||

O Formless Lord, Unstained, Unmarked
O Primal Being, Pure Lord, without beginning, self-created
Only fools claim to know the Secrets of God
His Secrets are not known to the Vedas ||15||

One who sets up a stone idol as God
Is a total fool; he does not know the difference
He keeps on calling Shiva the Great God
But he does not know the Secrets of the Formless Lord God ||16||

According to their own understanding
People describe God in their own ways
Your extent and limits cannot be known
How the universe was first created cannot be known ||17||

He has One Form, of Unparalleled Beauty
He appears as a beggar, or a king, at different places
He created life from eggs, from the womb, from sweat
He created nature's abundant vegetation ||18||

Sometimes, He sits joyfully as an Emperor
Sometimes, He sits as a Yogi, detached from all
The entire creation unfolds as His Wondrous Miracle
From the beginning, throughout the ages, He is Unchanging, Self-created ||19||

Now, O Lord, please give me Your Protection
Save my Sikhs, and destroy the non-believers
Destroy our enemies who engage in evil and wickedness
Destroy all the filthy evil-doers on the field of battle ||20||

O Wielder of the Sword, those who seek Your Sanctuary
May their enemies meet a terrible death
Those who fall at Your Feet, O Lord
Please release them from all suffering ||21||

Those who meditate on the Almighty Lord, even once
Death cannot even approach them
The Lord will totally protect them forever
And their troubles and enemies will be gone in an instant ||22||

When the Lord casts His Glance of Grace
They are instantly freed of all suffering
All worldly and spiritual powers come to them in their own homes
Their enemies shall not even be able to touch their shadows ||23||

Whoever remembers You, O Lord, even once
Shall be saved from the noose of death
That person who chants Your Name,
Shall be freed from poverty and the attacks of his enemies ||24||

O Wielder of the Sword, I seek Your Sanctuary
Please, give me Your Hand, and save me
Please be my Helper and Support in all places
Please protect me from the evil plots of my enemies |25||

Svaye

Since I have grasped hold of Your Lotus Feet, My eyes have not gazed upon any other. Many call You 'Ram', and 'Rehim', and read the Puranas and the Koran, but I do not follow the teachings of any one religion. The Simritees, the Shastras and the Vedas all speak of many Mysteries of God, But I do not know any of them. O Supreme Sword, please bless me with Your Mercy; It is not I who speak, but You who speaks through me.

Dohra

Having turned my back on all other doors, I have come to Your Door. Please help me, and protect my honor. Gobind Singh is Your slave.

Ramkali, from the Third Guru, Anand - The Song Of Bliss

One Universal Creator God. By The Grace Of The True Guru

One Creator of the One Creation. By The Grace Of The True Guru:
I am in ecstasy, O my Mother, for I have found my True Guru.
I have found the True Guru, with intuitive ease, and my mind vibrates with the music of bliss.
The jewelled melodies & their celestial harmonies have come to sing the Word of the Shabd.
The Lord dwells within the minds of those who sing the Shabd.
Says Nanak, I am in ecstasy, for I have found my True Guru. ||1||

O my mind, remain always with the Lord.
Remain always with the Lord, O my mind, and all sufferings will be forgotten.
He will accept you as His own, and all your affairs will be perfectly arranged.
Our Lord and Master is all-powerful to do all things, so forget Him not.
Says Nanak, O my mind, remain always with the Lord. ||2||

O my True Lord and Master, what is there which is not in Your celestial home?
Everything is in Your home; they receive, unto whom You give.
Constantly singing Your Praises and Glories, Your Name is enshrined in the mind.
The divine melody of the Shabd vibrates for those, within whose minds the Nam abides.
Says Nanak, O my True Lord and Master, what is there which is not in Your home? ||3||

The True Name is my only support.
The True Name is my only support; it satisfies all hunger.
It has brought peace and tranquility to my mind; it has fulfilled all my desires.
I am forever a sacrifice to the Guru, who possesses such glorious greatness.
Says Nanak, listen, O Saints; enshrine love for the Shabd.
The True Name is my only support. ||4||

The Panch (Panj) Shabd, the five primal sounds, vibrate in that blessed house.
In that blessed house, the Shabd vibrates; He infuses His almighty power into it.

Through You, we subdue the five demons of desire, and slay death, the torturer.
Those who have such pre-ordained destiny are attached to the Lord's Name.
Says Nanak, they are at peace, and the unstruck sound current vibrates within their homes. ||5||

Listen to the song of bliss, O most fortunate ones; all your longings shall be fulfilled.
I have obtained the Supreme Lord God, and all sorrows have been forgotten.
Pain, illness and suffering have departed, listening to the True Bani.
The Saints and their friends are in ecstasy, knowing the Perfect Guru.
Pure are the listeners, and pure are the speakers; the True Guru is all-pervading and permeating.
Prays Nanak, touching the Guru's Feet, the unstruck sound current of the celestial bugles vibrates and resounds. ||40||1||

Mundavani, from the Fifth Guru

Upon this Plate, three things have been placed: Truth, Contentment and Contemplation. The Ambrosial Nectar of the Nam, the Name of our Lord and Master, has been placed upon it as well; it is the Support of all. One who eats it and enjoys it shall be saved. This thing can never be forsaken; keep this always and forever in your mind. The dark world-ocean is crossed over, by grasping the Feet of the Lord; O Nanak, it is all the extension of God. ||1||

Slok, from the Fifth Guru

I have not appreciated what You have done for me, Lord; only You can make me worthy. I am unworthy - I have no worth or virtues at all. You have taken pity on me. You took pity on me, and blessed me with Your Mercy, and I have met the True Guru, my Friend. O Nanak, if I am blessed with the Nam, I live, and my body and mind blossom forth. ||1||

Pauri, from the Fifth Guru

O powerful God, You exist where none else does. You give protection even amidst the fire of the womb. On hearing Your Name, the messengers of death depart. With the help of the Shabd (divine hymn), one crosses the terrible, vast world ocean. Those who are thirsty for it drink the Divine Nectar. In the age of Kaliyug (Dark Age) the singing of God's praises is the act of highest virtue. God is kind to all and takes care of all in every moment. None come empty handed from Your door, who come with faith.

Slok, from the Fifth Guru

Remember the Guru within and utter His word with ears (while listening). One imbued with the True Guru gets a place in God's home. Nanak says, he to whom God gives this gift obtains the Divine Grace. Such ones are rare and emerge as pious.

Hymn from the Fifth Guru

The Protector Himself saves all. He causes us to fall at the feet of the Guru and fulfills the task. When He becomes merciful He does not forget the devotee. He provides means for the devotee to cross the world ocean by giving him the society of the True Saints. He destroys the non-believers and sinners in a moment. Nanak says, I take shelter of my master in my mind. By remembering Whom, bliss comes and all pains vanish. ||2||[157]

KIRTAN SOHILA

This *bani* is the night time prayer of the Sikhs and is spoken before going to sleep. It is a hymn of celebration; about both the bliss of Divine Union, as well as the pain of separation. *Guru Nanak, Guru Ram Das* and *Guru Arjun Dev* each contributed to this prayer. It is believed that chanting this mantra helps to relieve one from insomnia and provides protection from negativity.[158] **Kirtan** in this context means *song*; **Sohila** means *praise(s)*. *Kirtan Sohila* is a *Song of Praises*.[159]

Sohïla

Rag Gauri Dipaki Mehla Pehila (1)

Ek ong kar Satïgur prasad
Je gar kirat aki-ey kartey ka ho-ey bicharo
Tït gar gavau sohïla sïvrï-hu sirjan-haro ||1||

Tūm gavau mey-rey nirbao ka sohïla
Ha-o vari jït sohïley sada sūk ho-ey ||1|| Rahao

Nït nït jia-rey samali-an deyk-heyga dey-vanhar
Tey-rey daney kimat na pavey tïs datey kavan sūmar ||2||

Sambat saha lïkia mïl kar pavau teyl
Dey sajan asi sri-a jio hovey sahïb sio meyl ||3||

Gar Gar ey-ho pa-hūcha sad-rey nït pavan
Sadan-hara sïmri-ey Nanïk sey di-avan ||4||1||

Rag Asa Mehla Pehila (1)

Chia gar chia gur chia ūpdeys
Gur gur eyko veys aneyk ||1||
Baba jey gar kartey ki-rat ho-ey
So gar rak vada-i to-ey ||1|| Rahao

Vïsu-ey chasi-a gar-hia peh-ra tïti vari mau hoa
Sūraj eyko rūt aneyk
Nanïk kartey key key-tey veys ||2||2||

Rag Dhanasri Mehla Pehila (1)

Gagan mey tal rav chand di-pak
Baney tarika mandal janïk moti
Dūp mal-anlo pavan chavro
Karey sagal banra-ey fū-lant joti ||1||

132

Key-si arti ho-ey Bav kand-na teyri arti
Anhata sabd vajant bheyri ||1|| Rahao

Sahas tav nen nan nen heh to-hi
Ka-o sahas mūrït nana eyk to-hi
Sahas pad bïmal nan eyk pad gand bïn
Sahas tav gand ïv chalat mo-hi ||2||

Sab meh jot jot hey so-ey
Tïs dey chanan sab meh chanan ho-ey
Gur sak-hi jot pargat ho-ey
Jo tïs bavey so arti ho-ey ||3||

Har charn kaval makrand lob-hït
Mano andïno mo-hi ahi pi-asa
Kirpa jal de Nanïk sarïng kao
Ho-ey ja-tey tey-rey na-ey vasa ||4||3||

Rag Gauri Pūrbi Mehla Chauta (4)

Kam karod nagar ba-ho bari-a
Mïl sadhu kandal kanda hey
Pūrab lïkat lïkey gur pai-a man
Har lïv mandal manda hey ||1||
Kar sadhu anjūli pan vada hey
Kar dand-ūt pan vada hey ||1|| Rahao

Sakat har ras sad-na jania
Tïn antar ha-ūmey kanda hey
Jio jio cha-le chū-bey dūk pava-hi
Jamkal sa-he sir danda hey ||2||
Har jan har har nam samaney dūk
Janam maran bav kanda hey
Abïnasi purk pai-a parmey-sar
Ba-ho sob kand brah-manda hey ||3||

Ham gar-ib mas-kin parb tey-rey
Har rak rak vad vada hey
Han Nanïk nam ad-har teyk hey
Har namey hi sūk manda hey ||4||4||

Rag Gauri Pūrbi Mehla Panjva (5)

Kara-o bey-nanti sūn-hu mey-rey
Mita sant tahal ki bey-la
I-ha kat chal-hu har la-ha
Agey basan su-heyla ||1||

133

A-od gatey dïnas rey-narey
Man gur mïl kaj savarey ||1|| Rahao

Eh sansar bikar sansey me tari-o baram gi-ani
Jïsa-hi jaga-ey pi-avey eh ras akat kath tïn jani ||2||

Ja ka-o a-ey so-i bi-hajau har gūr tey ma-ne basey-ra
Nïj gar mahal pavu sūk se-jey ba-ur na ho-igo feyra ||3||

Antar-jami purk bi-datey sarda man ki pūrey
Nanïk dasi hey sūk magey moka-o kar santan ki dūrey ||4||5||

Song of Praises

Gauri Dipaki, from the First Guru

In that house where the Praises of the Creator are chanted and contemplated; In that house, sing Songs of Praise; Meditate and remember the Creator Lord. ||1||
Sing the Songs of Praise of my Fearless Lord. I am a sacrifice to that Song of Praise which brings eternal peace. ||1||Pause||

Day after day, He cares for His beings; the Great Giver watches over all. Your Gifts cannot be appraised; how can anyone compare to the Giver? ||2||

The day of my wedding is pre-ordained. Come, gather together and pour the oil over the threshold. My friends, give me your blessings, that I may merge with my Lord and Master. ||3||

Unto each and every home, into each and every heart, this summons is sent out; the call comes each and every day. Remember in meditation the One who summons us; O Nanak, that day is drawing near! ||4||1||

Asa, from the first Guru

There are six schools of philosophy, six teachers, and six sets of teachings. But the Teacher of teachers is the One, who appears in so many forms. ||1||
O Baba, that system in which the Praises of the Creator are sung; Follow that system, for in it rests true greatness. ||1||Pause||

The seconds, minutes and hours, days, weeks and months, and the various seasons originate from the One Sun; O Nanak, in just the same way, the many forms originate from the Creator. ||2||2||

Danasri, from the First Guru

Upon that cosmic plate of the sky is the sun and the moon is the lamp. The stars and their orbs are the studded pearls.
The fragrance of sandalwood in the air is the temple incense, and the wind is the fan. All the plants of the world are the altar flowers in offering to You, O Luminous Lord. ||1||
What a beautiful Arti, lamp-lit worship service this is! O Destroyer of Fear, this is Your Ceremony of Light. The Unstruck Sound-current of the Shabd is the vibration of the temple drums. ||1||Pause||

You have thousands of eyes, and yet You have no eyes. You have thousands of forms, and yet You do not have even one. You have thousands of Lotus Feet, and yet You do not have even one foot. You have no nose, but you have thousands of noses. This Play of Yours entrances me. ||2||
Amongst all is the Light; You are that Light. By this Illumination, that Light is radiant within all. Through the Guru's Teachings, the Light shines forth. That which is pleasing to Him is the lamp-lit worship service. ||3||

My mind is enticed by the honey-sweet Lotus Feet of the Lord. Day and night, I thirst for them. Bestow the Water of Your Mercy upon Nanak, the thirsty song-bird, so that he may come to dwell in Your Name. ||4||3||

Gauri Pūrbi, from the Fourth Guru

Lust and anger completely fill this village (body); These were broken into bits when I met with the Holy Saint. By pre-ordained destiny, I have met with the Guru. I have entered into the realm of the Lord's Love. ||1||
Greet the Holy Saint with your palms pressed together; this is an act of great merit. Bow down before Him; this is a virtuous action indeed. ||1||Pause||

The wicked shaktas, the faithless cynics, do not know the Taste of the Lord's Sublime Essence. The thorn of egotism is embedded deep within them. The more they walk away, the deeper it pierces them, and the more they suffer in pain, until finally, the Messenger of Death smashes his club against their heads. ||2||

The humble servants of the Lord are absorbed in the Name of the Lord, Har, Har. The pain of birth and the fear of death are eradicated. They have found the Imperishable Supreme Being, the Transcendent Lord God, and they receive great honor throughout all the worlds and realms. ||3||

I am poor and meek, God, but I belong to You! Save me; please save me, O Greatest of the Great! Servant Nanak takes the Sustenance and Support of the Nam. In the Name of the Lord, he enjoys celestial peace. ||4||4||

Gauri Pūrbi, from the Fifth Guru

Listen, my friends, I beg of you: now is the time to serve the Saints! In this world, earn the profit of the Lord's Name, and hereafter, you shall dwell in peace. ||1||
This life is diminishing, day and night. Meeting with the Guru, your affairs shall be resolved. ||1||Pause||

This world is engrossed in corruption and cynicism. Only those who know God are saved. Only those who are awakened by the Lord to drink in this Sublime Essence, come to know the Unspoken Speech of the Lord. ||2||

Purchase only that for which you have come into the world, and through the Guru, the Lord shall dwell within your mind. Within the home of your own inner being, you shall obtain the Mansion of the Lord's Presence with intuitive ease. You shall not be consigned again to the wheel of reincarnation. ||3||

O Inner-knower, Searcher of Hearts; O Primal Being, Architect of Destiny, please fulfill this yearning of my mind. Nanak, Your slave, begs for this happiness; Let me be the dust at the feet of the Saints. ||4||5||[160]

APPENDIX A

Recommended Listening Tools

This section was created in order to provide a **list of recommended recordings** for each of the mantras that appear in this manual so that one may have the benefit of listening and reading simultaneously. I have long found this to be the key to learning the sounds and eventually, memorizing mantras. For information on where to purchase audio recordings mentioned in this section, please see APPENDIX B on page 142.

IMPORTANT NOTE:
It is especially important in many meditations to use the correct rhythm of the chant and not just a beautiful musical version. For this reason, please refer to the KRI website as the default source for pronunciation as it contains the most precise versions. www.kundaliniresearchinstitute.org

Frequently Used Kundalini Yoga Mantras

Ong Namo Guru Deyv Namo (Adi Mantra)
  Kundalini Mantra Instruction by *Gurudass Kaur* (Tuning In & Individual Meditation Versions)
  Mantras of the Master by *Santokh Singh PhD* (Tuning In Version)
  Shashara by *Sada Sat Kaur* (Musical Version)
  Grace by *Snatam Kaur* (Musical Version)

Sat Nam
  Mantras of the Master by *Santokh Singh PhD* (Long Version)
  Deeply Relax and Meditate – Companion for Kundalini Yoga by *Shakta Kaur Khalsa* (Long Version)

Sa Ta Na Ma (Panj Shabd for Kirtan Kriya)
  Sa Ta Na Ma – 62 Minutes by *Snatam Kaur* (Chanted Version)
  Kundalini Mantra Instruction by *Gurudass Kaur* (Chanted Version)
  Mantras of the Master by *Santokh Singh PhD* (Chanted Version)

Aad Gurey Nameh (Mangalacharn Mantra)
  Kundalini Mantra Instruction by *Gurudass Kaur* (Chanted Version)
  Mantras of the Master by *Santokh Singh PhD* (Chanted Version)
  Prem by *Snatam Kaur* (Musical Version)
  The Guru Singh Experience Volume II by *Guru Singh* (Musical Version)

Long Time Sun
  Grace by *Snatam Kaur* (Musical Version)
  On This Day by *Hari Bhajan Kaur* (Musical Version)
  Cozy by *Shakta Kaur Khalsa* (Musical Version)

Aquarian Sadhana Mantras

Complete Sadhana Albums
  Raga Sadhana Volumes 1 or 2 by *Sangeet Kaur Khalsa*
  A Daily Practice by *Sat Kartar Kaur*
  African Dawn by *Siri Dharma Kaur*
  Grateful Ganesh by *Guru Ganesha Singh* (No long Ek-Ong-Kar)

Other Mantras from Kundalini Yoga

Aad Gurey Nameh (Mangalacharn Mantra)
> *Kundalini Mantra Instruction* by *Gurudass Kaur* (Chanted Version)
> *Mantras of the Master* by *Santokh Singh PhD* (Chanted Version)
> *Prem* by *Snatam Kaur* (Musical Version)
> *The Guru Singh Experience Volume II* by *Guru Singh* (Musical Version)

Aad Sach
> *Kundalini Mantra Instruction* by *Gurudass Kaur* (Chanted Version)
> *Naad Mantra* by *Guru Singh* (Chanted Version)
> *Green House* by *Gurunam* (Musical Version)

Aap Sahai Hoa
> *Naad Mantra* by *Guru Singh* (Chanted Version)
> *Game of Chants* by *Guru Singh* (Musical Version)
> *Circle of Light* by *Gurudass* (Musical Version)

Aadeys Tisey Aadeys
> *Prem* by *Snatam Kaur* (Musical Version)

Adi Mantra (For Individual Meditation)
> *Kundalini Mantra Instruction* by *Gurudass Kaur* (Chanted Version)
> *Mantras of the Master* by *Santokh Singh PhD* (Chanted Version)
> *Ignite Your Light* by *Satkirin Kaur Khalsa* (Musical Version)
> *Bringing Heaven To Earth* by *Tarn Taran Singh & Friends* (Musical Version)

Adi Shakti
> *Mantras of the Master* by *Santokh Singh PhD* (Chanted Version)
> *Angel's Waltz* by *Sada Sat Kaur* (Musical Version)
> *Pure Ganesh* by *Guru Ganesha Singh* (Musical Version)

Ajai Alai
> *Mantras of the Master* by *Santokh Singh PhD* (Chanted Version)
> *Shashara* by *Sada Sat Kaur* (Musical Version)
> *Ocean* by *Mirabai Ceiba* (Musical Version)

Akal
> *Kundalini Mantra Instruction* by *Gurudass Kaur* (Chanted Version)
> *Akal – Undying* by *Snatam Kaur* (Musical Version)

Akan Jor
> *Shanti* by *Snatam Kaur* (Musical Version)
> *From Fear to Love* by *Satya Singh Khalsa* (Musical Version)

Alak Baba Siri Chand Di-Rak
> *Mantras of the Master* by *Santokh Singh PhD* (Chanted Version)

Anand
> *Anand* by *Snatam Kaur* (Musical Version)

Anand Sahïb
> *Daily Banis* by *Amarjit Kaur* (Chanted Version)
> *Darsh Tere Ki Pyas* by *Bhai Harjinder Singh* (Musical Version)

Ang Sang Wahe Guru
> *Kundalini Mantra Instruction* by *Gurudass Kaur* (Chanted Version)
> *Mantras of the Master* by *Santokh Singh PhD* (Chanted Version)
> *Flow* by *Sat Kartar* (Musical Version)
> *Longing to Belong* by *Gurudass* (Musical Version)

Ant-na Sifti
>*Ocean* by *Mirabai Ceiba* (Musical Version)

Ardas Bahi
>*Kundalini Mantra Instruction* by *Gurudass Kaur* (Chanted Version)
>*Crimson Collection Volume 6 & 7* by *Singh Kaur* (Musical Version)
>*Liberations Door* by *Snatam Kaur & Guru Ganesha Singh* (Musical Version)
>*The Sweetest Nectar* by *Simrit Kaur* (Musical Version)

Aval Allah
>*Enchanted* by *Gurudass* (Musical Version)

Aaaa-Oooo-Ummm
>*Mantras of the Master* by *Santokh Singh PhD* (Chanted Version)

Ba-ota Karam
>*None (See Japji Sahib)*

Bolo Ram
>*Angel's Waltz* by *Sada Sat Kaur* (Musical Version)

Bole Sonihal – Deyh Shiva
>*None*

Bountiful, Blissful, Beautiful
>*Soul Songs* by *Bhajan Kaur* (Musical Version)
>*Pure Ganesh* by *Guru Ganesha Singh* (Musical Version on the Track *Ma*)

By Thy Grace
>*Grace* by *Snatam Kaur* (Musical Version)

Chakra Chihn
>*Shakti* by *Guru Shabad Singh Khalsa* (Musical Version)
>*Mangala Charan of Jaap Sahib* by *Sat Kirin Kaur* (Musical Version)

Charn Sat Sat
>*Liberations Door* by *Snatam Kaur & Guru Ganesha Singh* (Musical Version)

Chatr Chakr Varti
>*Kundalini Mantra Instruction* by *Gurudass Kaur* (Chanted Version)
>*Mantras of the Master* by *Santokh Singh PhD* (Chanted Version)
>*Lightness of Being* by *Sat Kirin Kaur* (Musical Version)
>*Kundalini Beat* by *Dev Suroop Kaur* (Musical Version)

Chardi Kala
>*Liberations Door* by *Snatam Kaur & Guru Ganesha Singh* (Musical Version)

Dhan Dhan Ram Das Guru
>*Mantras of the Master* by *Santokh Singh PhD* (Chanted Version)
>*Enchanted* by *Gurudass* (Musical Version)
>*Mother's Blessing* by *Snatam Kaur & Prabhu Nam Kaur* (Musical Version)
>*Naad Mantra* by *Guru Singh* (Chanted Version)

Dharti Hae (Isht Shodhana Mantra)
>*Isht Shodhana Mantra* by *Gurucharan S Khalsa PhD* (Chanted Version)
>*Silent Moonlight Meditation* by *Gurunam Singh* (Musical Version)

Duk Par Har
>*None (See Japji Sahib)*

Ek Ong Kar-ah (Laya Yoga Mantra)
Kundalini Mantra Instruction by *Gurudass Kaur* (Chanted Version)
Mantras of the Master by *Santokh Singh PhD* (Chanted Version)
Listen by *Sat Kartar* (Musical Version)

Ek Ong Kar Sat Gur Prasad (Sïri Mantra)
Kundalini Mantra Instruction by *Gurudass Kaur* (Chanted Version)
Mantras of the Master by *Santokh Singh PhD* (Chanted Version)
Listen by *Sat Kartar* (Musical Version)

Eterno Sol (Long Time Sun – Spanish)
Ocean by *Mirabai Ceiba* (Musical Version)

Ganapati Mantra (Panj Shabd with Siri Gaitri Mantra)
Kundalini Mantra Instruction by *Gurudass Kaur* (Chanted Version)
Mantras of the Master by *Santokh Singh PhD* (Chanted Version)

Gobinda Hari
Prem by *Snatam Kaur* (Musical Version)
Angel's Waltz by *Sada Sat Kaur* (Musical Version)

Gobindey Mukandey
Kundalini Mantra Instruction by *Gurudass Kaur* (Chanted Version)
Mantras of the Master by *Santokh Singh PhD* (Chanted Version)
Enchanted by *Gurudass* (Musical Version)
Shashara by *Sada Sat Kaur* (Musical Version)

God And Me
Destiny by *Yogi Bhajan* (Chanted Version)

Guru Deyv Mata
Nectar of the Name by *Sat Purkh Kaur Khalsa* (Musical Version)

Guru Ram Das Chant
Flores by *Mirabai Ceiba* (Musical Version)
Enchanted by *Gurudass* (Musical Version)
Mantra Masala by *Sada Sat Kaur* (Musical Version)
Heaven's Touch by *Gurunam* (Musical Version)
Angel's Waltz by *Sada Sat Kaur* (Musical Version)
Shanti by *Snatam Kaur* (Musical Version)
The Miracle Mantra of Guru Ram Das by *Gurucharan S Khalsa PhD* (2 Musical Versions)

Guru Ram Das Rako Sarana-i
Anand by *Snatam Kaur* (Musical Version)
Song of the Soul by *Hari Bhajan Kaur & Sat Hari Singh* (Musical Version)

Guru Sat Guru
None

Ham Dam Har Har
From Fear to Love by *Satya Singh Khalsa* (Musical Version)

Ha-mi Ham Brahm Ham
Kundalini Mantra Instruction by *Gurudass Kaur* (Chanted Version)
Mantras of the Master by *Santokh Singh PhD* (Chanted Version)
Humee Hum & Tranquility by *Niranjan K Khalsa* (Musical Version)
Game of Chants by *Guru Singh* (Musical Version)
The Guru Singh Experience Volume II by *Guru Singh* (Musical Version)

Ha-mi Ham Tu-mi Tum
Kundalini Mantra Instruction by *Gurudass Kaur* (Chanted Version)
Mantras of the Master by *Santokh Singh PhD* (Chanted Version)

Har

     Tantric Har & Har Har Wahe Guru by *Simran Kaur Khalsa* (Musical Version)

Har Gobind Mahan Hae

     Asankh Nav by *Gurudass* (Musical Version)

Har Har Har Amritsar

     Flow by *Sat Kartar* (Musical Version)

Har Har Har Har Gobindey (Guru Gairti Mantra with 4 Hars)

     Kundalini Mantra Instruction by *Gurudass Kaur* (Chanted Version)

     Mantras of the Master by *Santokh Singh PhD* (Chanted Version)

     Mantra Masala by *Sada Sat Kaur* (Musical Version)

     Dubiquity by *Aurora* (Musical Version)

Har Har Har Har Harinam

     Pure Ganesh by *Guru Ganesha Singh* (Musical Version)

Har Har Mukandey

     Kundalini Mantra Instruction by *Gurudass Kaur* (Chanted Version)

     Mantras of the Master by *Santokh Singh PhD* (Chanted Version)

Har Har Ram Das Guru Hae

     Liberations Door by *Snatam Kaur & Guru Ganesha Singh* (Musical Version)

Har Har Wahe Guru

     Kundalini Mantra Instruction by *Gurudass Kaur* (Chanted Version)

     Mantras of the Master by *Santokh Singh PhD* (Chanted Version)

     Har Har Wahe Guru by *WAH!* (Musical Version)

Har Harey Hari Wahe Guru

     Kundalini Mantra Instruction by *Gurudass Kaur* (Chanted Version)

     Mantras of the Master by *Santokh Singh PhD* (Chanted Version)

     Tantric Har & Har Har Wahe Guru by *Simran Kaur Khalsa* (Musical Version)

     Longing To Belong by *Gurudass* (Musical Version)

Har Hari

     None

Har Ji

     Har Ji – Mirror of The Soul by *Ram Singh* (Musical Version)

Har Ka Nam

     None

Har Singh Nar Singh

     Mantras of the Master by *Santokh Singh PhD* (Chanted Version)

     Adhara by *Nirinjan Kaur* (Musical Version)

Har Wahe Guru Sat Nam Har Hari

     The Flow of Naam by *Gurunam* (Musical Version)

Hari Nam Sat Nam

     Mantras of the Master by *Santokh Singh PhD* (Chanted Version)

I Am I Am

     Flow by *Sat Kartar* (Musical Version)

     Game of Chants by *Guru Singh* (Musical Version)

     Sounds of the Ether by *Gurunam* (Musical Version)

I Am Happy I Am Good
> *Feeling Good Today* by *Snatam Kaur* (Musical Version)
> I Am The Light Of My Soul
> *Feeling Good Today* by *Snatam Kaur* (Musical Version)
> *I Am the Light of The Soul* by *Bibi Bhani Kaur* (Musical Version)
> *Adhara* by *Nirinjan Kaur* (Musical Version)

Jap Man Sat Nam
> *Mantras of the Master* by *Santokh Singh PhD* (Chanted Version)
> *Anand* by *Snatam Kaur* (Musical Version)

Jap Sahib
> *Jaap Sahib* by *Prof. Sat Nam Singh* (Musical Version)
> *Daily Banis* by *Amarjit Kaur* (Chanted Version)
> *Bani Pro 1* by *Rajnarind Kaur* (Chanted Version)

Japji Sahib
> *Japji Sahib* by *Bhai Balbir Singh* (Chanted Version)
> *Daily Banis* by *Amarjit Kaur* (Chanted Version)
> *Japji Sahib* by *Guru Raj Kaur* (Chanted, Musical & Tantric Versions)
> *Japji Sahib* by *Baba Singh* (Tantric Version)
> *Japji Sahib* by *Prof. Sat Nam Singh* (Musical Version)

Jei Te Gang
> *Silent Moonlight Meditation* by *Gurunam Singh* (Musical Version)
> *Adhara* by *Nirinjan Kaur* (Musical Version)

Jin Prema Kio
> *Prem* by *Snatam Kaur* (Musical Version)

Kal Akal
> *Mantras of the Master* by *Santokh Singh PhD* (Chanted Version)
> *Dubiquity* by *Aurora* (Musical Version)
> *Pavan Pavan* by *Guru Shabad Singh Khalsa* (Musical Version)

Kauri Kriya Mantra (Sargam, Panj Shabd and Siri Gaitri Mantra)
> *Mantras of the Master* by *Santokh Singh PhD* (Chanted Version)

Kirtan Sohila
> *Daily Banis* by *Amarjit Kaur* (Chanted Version)
> *Bani Pro 1* by *Rajnarind Kaur* (Chanted Version)

Long Time Sun
> *Grace* by *Snatam Kaur* (Musical Version)
> *On This Day* by *Hari Bhajan Kaur* (Musical Version)
> *Cozy* by *Shakta Kaur Khalsa* (Musical Version)

Maaa
> *Pure Ganesh* by *Guru Ganesha Singh* (Musical Version)
> *Silent Moonlight Meditation* by *Gurunam Singh* (Musical Version)

Maha Mrityunjai Mantra
> *Mrityunjaya Mantra – Sanskrit Chant* by *Manorama* (Chanted Version)
> *Mantram – Chant of India* by *Ravi Shankar* (Chanted Version)
> *Maha Mrityunjai Mantra* by *Alka Yagnik* (Musical Version)

Mangala Saj Beya
> *Shabd Volume I* by *Satkirin Kaur Khalsa* (Musical Version)

Me Within Me
> *None*

Mere Man Lochey
>	*Nectar of the Name* by *Purkh Kaur Khalsa* (Musical Version)
>	*Universal Prayer* by *Sat Kirin Kaur* (Musical Version)

Mul Mantra
>	*Kundalini Mantra Instruction* by *Gurudass Kaur* (Chanted Version)
>	*Mantras of the Master* by *Santokh Singh PhD* (Chanted Version)
>	*Anand* by *Snatam Kaur* (Musical Version)
>	*Shashara* by *Sada Sat Kaur* (Musical Version)
>	*Har Ji – Mirror of The Soul* by *Ram Singh* (Musical Version)
>	*Celebration* by *Carioca* (Musical Version)
>	*Power Mantras* by *Guru Ganesha Singh* (Musical Version)
>	*Longing To Belong* by *Gurudass* (Musical Version)
>	*Crimson Collection Volume I & II* by *Singh Kaur* (Musical Version)
>	*Mul Mantra & Wahe Guru* by *Simran Kaur Khalsa* (Tantric Version)

On This Day
>	*On This Day* by *Hari Bhajan Kaur* (Musical Version)
>	*Deeply Relax and Meditate – Companion for Kundalini Yoga* by *Shakta Kaur Khalsa* (Musical Version)

Ong
>	*Kundalini Mantra Instruction* by *Gurudass Kaur* (Chanted Version)
>	*Mantras of the Master* by *Santokh Singh PhD* (Chanted Version)
>	*Enchanted* by *Gurudass* (Musical Version on the Track *Ek Ong Kar*)

Ong Kar Nirankar
>	*Lovingly* by *Gurudass Kaur* (Musical Version)

Ong Namo Guru Deyv Namo (Adi Mantra)
>	*Kundalini Mantra Instruction* by *Gurudass Kaur* (Tuning In & Individual Meditation Versions)
>	*Mantras of the Master* by *Santokh Singh PhD* (Tuning In Version)
>	*Shashara* by *Sada Sat Kaur* (Musical Version)
>	*Grace* by *Snatam Kaur* (Musical Version)

Ong Sohang
>	*Kundalini Mantra Instruction* by *Gurudass Kaur* (Chanted Version)
>	*Mantras of the Master* by *Santokh Singh PhD* (Chanted Version)
>	*Shanti* by *Snatam Kaur* (Musical Version)
>	Parameysarey
>	*Anand* by *Snatam Kaur* (Musical Version)

Pavan Guru
>	*Kundalini Mantra Instruction* by *Gurudass Kaur* (Chanted Version)
>	*Mantras of the Master* by *Santokh Singh PhD* (Chanted Version)
>	*Lovingly* by *Gurudass Kaur* (Musical Version)
>	*Pavan Pavan* by *Guru Shabad Singh Khalsa* (Musical Version)

People Of Love
>	*Celebrate Peace* by *Snatam Kaur* (Musical Version)

Prana Apana Sushumna
>	*None*

Ra Ma Da Sa (Siri Gaitri Mantra)
>	*Kundalini Mantra Instruction* by *Gurudass Kaur* (Chanted Version)
>	*Mantras of the Master* by *Santokh Singh PhD* (Chanted Version)
>	*Grace* by *Snatam Kaur* (Musical Version)
>	*Angel's Waltz* by *Sada Sat Kaur* (Musical Version)
>	*Lovingly* by *Gurudass Kaur* (Musical Version)

Ra Ma
> *Mantras of the Master* by *Santokh Singh PhD* (Chanted Version)

Ra Ra Ra Ra Ma Ma Ma Ma
> *Kundalini Mantra Instruction* by *Gurudass Kaur* (Chanted Version)
> *Mantras of the Master* by *Santokh Singh PhD* (Chanted Version)
> *Longing To Belong* by *Gurudass* (Musical Version)

Ra-ke Rakana Har
> *Kundalini Mantra Instruction* by *Gurudass Kaur* (Chanted Version)
> *Mantras of the Master* by *Santokh Singh PhD* (Chanted Version)
> *Rakhe Rakhan Har – 31 Minutes* by *Snatam Kaur* (Musical Version)
> *Radiance – Music For Morning Meditation* by *Dev Suroop Kaur* (Musical Version)
> *Mountain Sadhana* by *Mirabai Ceiba* (Musical Version)
> *Beautiful Sadhana* by *Gurutrang Singh* (Musical Version)
> *Aquarian Sadhana Mantras* by *Nirinjan Kaur* (Musical Version)

Ram Ram Hari Ram
> *Meditations Transformation – Experience & Project* by *Snatam Kaur* (Musical Version)

Rehiras Sahib
> *Daily Banis* by *Amarjit Kaur* (Chanted Version)
> *Bani Pro 1* by *Rajnarind Kaur* (Chanted Version)

Rey Man Shabd
> *Bound Lotus Companion CD* by *Snatam Kaur* (Chanted & Musical Versions)
> *Adhara* by *Nirinjan Kaur* (Musical Version)

Sa Rey Sa Sa
> *Kundalini Mantra Instruction* by *Gurudass Kaur* (Chanted Version)
> *Mantras of the Master* by *Santokh Singh PhD* (Chanted Version)
> *Sa Re Sa Sa* by *Guru Shabad Singh Khalsa* (Musical Version)
> *Ocean* by *Mirabai Ceiba* (Musical Version)

Sa Ta Na Ma (Panj Shabd for Kirtan Kriya)
> *Sa Ta Na Ma – 62 Minutes* by *Snatam Kaur* (Chanted Version)
> *Kundalini Mantra Instruction* by *Gurudass Kaur* (Chanted Version)
> *Mantras of the Master* by *Santokh Singh PhD* (Chanted Version)

Sat Guru Ho-ey Dyal
> *Mother's Blessing* by *Snatam Kaur & Prabhu Nam Kaur* (Musical Version)

Sat Kartar
> *Flow* by *Sat Kartar* (Musical Version)

Sat Nam
> *Mantras of the Master* by *Santokh Singh PhD* (Long Version)
> *Deeply Relax and Meditate – Companion for Kundalini Yoga* by *Shakta Kaur Khalsa* (Long Version)
> *Grace* by *Snatam Kaur* (Musical Version on the Track *Long Time Sun*)

Sat Nam Wahe Guru
> *Kundalini Mantra Instruction* by *Gurudass Kaur* (Chanted Version)
> *Mantras of the Master* by *Santokh Singh PhD* (Chanted Version)
> *Crimson Collection Volume III* by *Singh Kaur* (Musical Version Variation)

Sat Narayan
> *Kundalini Mantra Instruction* by *Gurudass Kaur* (Chanted Version)
> *Mantras of the Master* by *Santokh Singh PhD* (Chanted Version)
> *Livelight* by *Akyanna* (Musical Version)
> *Longing To Belong* by *Gurudass* (Musical Version)
> *Joy Is Now* by *Guru Ganesha Singh* (Musical Version)

Sat Siri Siri Akal
>*Kundalini Mantra Instruction* by *Gurudass Kaur* (Chanted Version)
>*Mantras of the Master* by *Santokh Singh PhD* (Chanted Version)
>*Shashara* by *Sada Sat Kaur* (Musical Version)
>*Dubiquity* by *Aurora* (Musical Version)
>*Nierika: The Gateway* by *Dharm Khalsa* (Musical Version)
>*Mountain Sadhana* by *Mirabai Ceiba* (Musical Version)

Shabd Hazarey
>*Daily Banis* by *Amarjit Kaur* (Chanted Version)
>*Bani Pro 1* by *Rajnarind Kaur* (Chanted Version)

So Purkh
>*So Purkh – That Primal God* by *Nirinjan Kaur* (Chanted Version)
>*So Purkh – That Primal God* by *Satkirin Kaur Khalsa* (Chanted Version)

Sochey Soch
>*Mantra Masala* by *Sada Sat Kaur* (Musical Version)

Soi Sunandari
>*Mother's Blessing* by *Snatam Kaur & Prabhu Nam Kaur* (Musical Version)

Suni-ey
>*Shanti* by *Snatam Kaur* (Musical Version)
>*Seasons of the Soul* by *Prabhu Nam Kaur* (Musical Version)
>*11* by *Ram Singh* (Musical Version)

Tav Prasad Svaye
>*Daily Banis* by *Amarjit Kaur* (Chanted Version)
>*Bani Pro 1* by *Rajnarind Kaur* (Chanted Version)

Teri Mehr Da Bolna
>*Meditations Transformation: Connect & Heal* by *Snatam Kaur* (Musical Version)

Triple Mantra
>*Mantras of the Master* by *Santokh Singh PhD* (Chanted Version)
>*Triple Mantra* by *Gurunam* (Chanted Version)
>*Adhara* by *Nirinjan Kaur* (Musical Version)

Wahe Guru
>*Kundalini Mantra Instruction* by *Gurudass Kaur* (Chanted Version)
>*Mantras of the Master* by *Santokh Singh PhD* (Chanted Version)
>*Tantric Wahe Guru* by *Snatam Kaur* (Tantric Version)
>*Mool Mantra & Wahe Guru* by *Simran Kaur Khalsa* (Musical Version)
>*Ignite Your Light* by *Satkirin Kau Khalsar* (Musical Version)
>*Lovingly* by *Gurudass Kaur* (Musical Version)
>*Enchanted* by *Gurudass* (Musical Version)

Wahe Guru Wahe Jio
>*Kundalini Mantra Instruction* by *Gurudass Kaur* (Chanted Version)
>*Bilssful Spirit* by *Gurunam* (Musical Version)
>*Mountain Sadhana* by *Mirabai Ceiba* (Musical Version)
>*Nierika: The Gateway* by *Dharm Khalsa* (Musical Version)
>*Prem* by *Snatam Kaur* (Musical Version)
>*Sadhana Rocks* by *Mata Mandir Singh* (Musical Version)

Wa Wa Hey Hey
>*Kundalini Mantra Instruction* by *Gurudass Kaur* (Chanted Version)

Wa Yanti
> *Kundalini Mantra Instruction* by *Gurudass Kaur* (Chanted Version)
> *Mantras of the Master* by *Santokh Singh PhD* (Chanted Version)
> *Aquarian Sadhana* by *Aurora* (Musical Version)
> *Game of Chants* by *Guru Singh* (Musical Version)
> *Mantra Masala* by *Sada Sat Kaur* (Musical Version)

We Are Peace
> *Celebrate Peace* by *Snatam Kaur* (Musical Version)

Sacred Nitnem

Japji Sahib
> *Japji Sahib* by *Bhai Balbir Singh* (Chanted Version)
> *Daily Banis* by *Amarjit Kaur* (Chanted Version)
> *Japji Sahib* by *Guru Raj Kaur* (Chanted, Musical & Tantric Versions)
> *Japji Sahib* by *Baba Singh* (Tantric Version)
> *Sahib* by *Prof. Sat Nam Singh* (Musical Version)

Jap Sahib
> *Jaap Sahib* by *Prof. Sat Nam Singh* (Musical Version)
> *Daily Banis* by *Amarjit Kaur* (Chanted Version)
> *Bani Pro 1* by *Rajnarind Kaur* (Chanted Version)

Shabd Hazarey
> *Daily Banis* by *Amarjit Kaur* (Chanted Version)
> *Bani Pro 1* by *Rajnarind Kaur* (Chanted Version)

Tav Prasad Svaye
> *Daily Banis* by *Amarjit Kaur* (Chanted Version)
> *Bani Pro 1* by *Rajnarind Kaur* (Chanted Version)

Anand Sahïb
> *Daily Banis* by *Amarjit Kaur* (Chanted Version)
> *Bani Pro 1* by *Rajnarind Kaur* (Chanted Version)
> *Darsh Tere Ki Pyas* by *Bhai Harjinder Singh* (Musical Version)

Rehiras Sahib
> *Daily Banis* by *Amarjit Kaur* (Chanted Version)
> *Bani Pro 1* by *Rajnarind Kaur* (Chanted Version)

Kirtan Sohila
> *Daily Banis* by *Amarjit Kaur* (Chanted Version)
> *Bani Pro 1* by *Rajnarind Kaur* (Chanted Version)

APPENDIX B

Where to Find Kundalini Yoga Mantra Music

Purchasing Kundalini Yoga music is highly recommended (rather than copying from others or searching for free downloads) for two reasons: #1 it is the honest way to obtain it; #2 if we want artists to continue to create new and unique recordings of Kundalini Yoga mantras, it is in our best interest to support them by paying for it. Here is a list of websites from where you can find recordings of the mantras listed within this manual.

Yoga Tech – www.yogatech.com
White Swan Music – www.whiteswanmusic.com
Ancient Healing Ways – www.a-healing.com
The Source – thesource.kriteachings.org
Ancient Healing Ways – http://www.a-healing.com

Kundalini Yoga Resources

Kundalini Research Institute – www.kriteachings.org
This website includes many printable downloads of kriyas and meditations, some videos of classes, a listening pronunciation guide for many mantras, information on The Aquarian Training Institute including a worldwiode listing of Level One Teacher Training Courses and Level Two Courses and an online store with books, DVDs and CDs.

Yogi Bhajan – www.yogibhajan.org
International Kundalini Yoga Teachers Associaiton – www.kundaliniyoga.com
This site has a searchable worldwide listing of accredited Kundalini Yoga Level One and Two Teachers and Level One Teacher Trainers.

3HO – www.3ho.org
This site includes information on the Summer and Winter Solstice Celebrations.

White Tantric Yoga – www.whitetantricyoga.com
This site includes a listing and contact information for worldwide White Tantric Yoga Courses.

REFERENCES

[1] Yogi Bhajan, Ph.D., (2003) *The Aquarian Teacher: KRI International Kundalini Yoga Teacher Training Level I.* (p. 78). Kundalini Research Institute.

[2] Score re-created by "L" based on illustrations that appear in all KRI Kundalini Yoga as Taught by Yogi Bhajan® manuals.

[3] Yogi Bhajan, Ph.D., (2003) *The Aquarian Teacher: KRI International Kundalini Yoga Teacher Training Level I.* (pp. 425-6). Kundalini Research Institute.

[4] Yogi Bhajan, Ph.D., (2003) *The Aquarian Teacher: KRI International Kundalini Yoga Teacher Training Level I.* (pp. 425-6). Kundalini Research Institute.

[5] Yogi Bhajan, Ph.D., (2003) *The Aquarian Teacher: KRI International Kundalini Yoga Teacher Training Level I.* (p. 82). Kundalini Research Institute.

[6] Kaur, Gurudass. Phone Interview. April 2010.

[7] Heron, Mike. (1968). *A Very Cellular Song* [Recorded by The Incredible String Band]. On the album *The Hangmans' Beautiful Daughter.*

[8] Yogi Bhajan, Ph.D., (2003) *The Aquarian Teacher: KRI International Kundalini Yoga Teacher Training Level I.* (pp. 152-3). Kundalini Research Institute.

[9] Yogi Bhajan, Ph.D., (2003) *The Aquarian Teacher: KRI International Kundalini Yoga Teacher Training Level I.* (p. 84). Kundalini Research Institute.

[10] Yogi Bhajan, Ph.D., (2003) *The Aquarian Teacher: KRI International Kundalini Yoga Teacher Training Level I.* (p. 152). Kundalini Research Institute.

[11] Yogi Bhajan, Ph.D., (2003) *The Aquarian Teacher: KRI International Kundalini Yoga Teacher Training Level I.* (p. 87). Kundalini Research Institute.

[12] Yogi Bhajan, Ph.D., (2003) *The Aquarian Teacher: KRI International Kundalini Yoga Teacher Training Level I.* (p. 152). Kundalini Research Institute.

[13] Yogi Bhajan, Ph.D., (2003) *The Aquarian Teacher: KRI International Kundalini Yoga Teacher Training Level I.* (p. 87). Kundalini Research Institute.

[14] Harbans Singh Doabia (2005), *Sacred Nitnem* (26th ed.). (p. 249) Amritsar, India: Singh Brothers Publishers. Translation appears with Permission from Singh Brothers Publishers.

[15] Yogi Bhajan, Ph.D., (2003) *The Aquarian Teacher: KRI International Kundalini Yoga Teacher Training Level I.* (p. 86). Kundalini Research Institute.

[16] Yogi Bhajan, Ph.D., (2003) *The Aquarian Teacher: KRI International Kundalini Yoga Teacher Training Level I.* (p. 87). Kundalini Research Institute.

[17] Yogi Bhajan, Ph.D., (2003) *The Aquarian Teacher: KRI International Kundalini Yoga Teacher Training Level I.* (p. 84). Kundalini Research Institute.

[18] Yogi Bhajan, Ph.D., (1999) *Kundalini Yoga Guidelines for Sadhana (Daily Practice).* (pp. 109-10). Española, New Mexico, USA: Kundalini Research Institute.

[19] Yogi Bhajan, Ph.D., (2003) *The Aquarian Teacher: KRI International Kundalini Yoga Teacher Training Level I.* (p. 82). Kundalini Research Institute

[20] Ibid

[21] Ibid

[22] Ibid

[23] Yogi Bhajan, Ph.D., (2003) *The Aquarian Teacher: KRI International Kundalini Yoga Teacher Training Level I.* (pp. 413-4). Kundalini Research Institute.

[24] Ibid

[25] Ibid

[26] Yogi Bhajan, Ph.D., (2003) *The Aquarian Teacher: KRI International Kundalini Yoga Teacher Training Level I.* (p. 82). Kundalini Research Institute.

[27] Yogi Bhajan, Ph.D., (2003) *The Aquarian Teacher: KRI International Kundalini Yoga Teacher Training Level I.* (p. 83). Kundalini Research Institute.

[28] SSS Harbhajan Singh Khalsa (Yogi Bhajan). Gurdwara Lecture. Akal Takhat and Deathlessness. 06 July 1989.

[29] Kaur, Ramdesh. Mantra for Protection Against Psychic Attack: Baba Siri Chand. 07 October 2010. <http://www.spiritvoyage.com/blog/index.php/mantra-for-protection-against-psychic-attack/>

[30] Anand Sahib. (09 May 2010). Retrieved on 10 Feb 2011 from <http://www.sikhiwiki.org/index.php/Anand_sahib>

[31] Yogi Bhajan, Ph.D., (2003) *The Aquarian Teacher: KRI International Kundalini Yoga Teacher Training Level I.* (p. 82). Kundalini Research Institute.

[32] Ibid

[33] Dipti. Aval Allah Noor Upaaya. (20 Jan 2008). Retrieved on 10 Feb 2011 from <http://aashiyaana.blogspot.com/2008/01/aval-allah-noor-upaaya.html>

[34] Yogi Bhajan, Ph.D., (2003) *The Aquarian Teacher: KRI International Kundalini Yoga Teacher Training Level I.* (p. 445). Kundalini Research Institute.

[35] Swami Chidanand Saraswati (Muniji), (2005) *Holy Days, A Year of Spiritual Celebration.* (p. 17). London: Garavi Gujarat Press.

[36] Khalsa, Guruprem Kaur and Khalsa, Atma Singh, from the Teachings of Yogi Bhajan, Ph.D. (2000). *A Year with the Master.* (p.101). Española, NM, USA: Yoga Gems.

[37] Yogi Bhajan, Ph.D., (2003) *The Aquarian Teacher: KRI International Kundalini Yoga Teacher Training Level I.* (p. 83). Kundalini Research Institute.

[38] Ibid

[39] Kaur, Snatam. "By Thy Grace". Grace. Spirit Voyage Music, 2004. CD. Lyrics appear with permission from Snatam Kaur.

[40] Raj Karega Khalsa Network. Jaap Sahib Line by Line Translation. Retrieved 11 Feb 2011 from
    <http://wn.com/Jaap_Sahib__Line_By_Line_Translation>

[41] Singh Aulakh, Ph. D., Dr. Ajit, (2000) *The Holy Sukhmaneee Sahib 8th Edition.* (p. 163). Amritsar, India: Publisher B. Chattar Singh Jiwan Singh.

[42] Singh Doabia, Harbans, (2005) *Sacred Nitnem 26th Edition.* (p.143). Amritsar, India: Singh Brothers. Translation appears with permission from Singh Brothers Publishing.

[43] Yogi Bhajan, Ph.D., (2003) *The Aquarian Teacher: KRI International Kundalini Yoga Teacher Training Level I.* (p. 83). Kundalini Research Institute.

[44] Chardi Kala. (2009). Retrieved on 10 February 2011 from
    <http://www.sikh.net/sikhism/chardikala.htm>

[45] SSS Harbhajan Singh Khalsa (Yogi Bhajan). Class Lecture. Cherdi Kala – Continuous Resurrection. 19 November 1989.

[46] Singh Ph.D., Santokh. "Dhan Dhan Ram Das Gur" (Track 15). Mantras of The Master. Kundalini Toolbox. 2008.

[47] Yogi Bhajan, Ph.D., (2003) *The Aquarian Teacher: KRI International Kundalini Yoga Teacher Training Level I.* (p. 83). Kundalini Research Institute.

[48] Khalsa Ph.D., Gurucharan S. "Lecture". Isht Shodhana Mantra Kriya. Miracle Mantra Series 1 Volume 2. Kundalini Research Institute. 2008. CD.

[49] Ibid

[50] Yogi Bhajan, Ph.D., (2003) *The Aquarian Teacher: KRI International Kundalini Yoga Teacher Training Level I.* (p. 427). Kundalini Research Institute.

[51] Ibid

[52] Swami Muktibodhananda, (2005) *Hatha Yoga Pradipika.* (p.619). Bihar, India: Yoga Publications Trust.

[53] Yogi Bhajan, Ph.D., (2003) *The Aquarian Teacher: KRI International Kundalini Yoga Teacher Training Level I.* (p. 84). Kundalini Research Institute.

[54] Ibid

[55] Yogi Bhajan, Ph.D., (1999) *Kundalini Yoga Guidelines for Sadhana (Daily Practice).* (pp. 71). Española, New Mexico, USA: Kundalini Research Institute

[56] Ibid

[57] Heron, Mike. (1968). *A Very Cellular Song* [Recorded by The Incredible String Band]. On the album *The Hangmans' Beautiful Daughter.*

[58] Khalsa, Harijot Kaur, (2001) *Self-Knowledge: Kundalini Yoga as Taught by Yogi Bhajan.* (p. 20). Kundalini Research Institute.

[59] Ibid

[60] Yogi Bhajan, Ph.D., (2003) *The Aquarian Teacher: KRI International Kundalini Yoga Teacher Training Level I.* (p. 84). Kundalini Research Institute.

[61] Bhajan, Yogi. "Me and God are One". Destiny. Kundalini Research Institute, 2005. CD.

[62] Khalsa, Guruprem Kaur and Khalsa, Atma Singh, from the Teachings of Yogi Bhajan, Ph.D. (2000). *A Year with the Master.* (p.103). Española, NM, USA: Yoga Gems.

[63] SSS Harbhajan Singh Khalsa (Yogi Bhajan). (2011). Air Tattva: The 2011 Global Meditation. Retrieved on 13 Feb 2011 from
    <https://docs.google.com/viewer?url=http://www.3ho.org/donations/images/air-tattva-instructions.pdf>

[64] Kaur, Snatam, Guru Ram Das Raakho Sarana-ee. (2006). Retrieved on 12 Feb 2011 from
    <http://www.snatamkaur.com/web7.html>

[65] Gur Satgur Ka Jo Sikh Akhai. Retrieved on 12 Feb 2011 from
    <http://www.sikhphilosophy.net/gurmat-vichaar/14247-gur-satgur-ka-jo-sikh-akhai.html >

[66] SSS Harbhajan Singh Khalsa (Yogi Bhajan). (1983). *Kundalini Yoga for Youth & Joy.* (p.57). Eugene: 3HO Transcripts.

[67] Yogi Bhajan, Ph.D., (2003) *The Aquarian Teacher: KRI International Kundalini Yoga Teacher Training Level I.* (p. 85). Kundalini Research Institute.

[68] SSS Harbhajan Singh Khalsa (Yogi Bhajan). (2013). 2013 First Sutra 40 Day Sadhana. Retrieved on 14 Mar 2014 from
    < http://www.3ho.org/events/global-meditations/2013-first-sutra-40-day-sadhana>

[69] SSS Harbhajan Singh Khalsa (Yogi Bhajan). Class Lecture. 1983.

[70] Yogi Bhajan, Ph.D., (2003) *The Aquarian Teacher: KRI International Kundalini Yoga Teacher Training Level I.* (p. 85). Kundalini Research Institute.

[71] Ibid

[72] Karan. (26 July 2009). Sunder Singh's Contribution to Snatam Kaur's New Release Liberation's Door. Retrieved 11 Feb 2011 from
    <http://www.spiritvoyage.com/blog/index.php/sunder-singhs-contribution-to-snatam-kaurs-new-release-liberations-door/>

[73] Yogi Bhajan, Ph.D., (2003) *The Aquarian Teacher: KRI International Kundalini Yoga Teacher Training Level I.* (p. 85). Kundalini Research Institute.

[74] Yogi Bhajan, Ph.D., (2003) *The Aquarian Teacher: KRI International Kundalini Yoga Teacher Training Level I.* (p. 84). Kundalini Research Institute.

[75] SSS Harbhajan Singh Khalsa (Yogi Bhajan). Class Lecture. Guru Nanak's Treasure Meditation. 11 Feb 1978. Meditation information can be retrieved from
    <http://www.dasvandh.org/meditations/guru-nanaks-treasure-meditation>

[76] Ibid

[77] SSS Harbhajan Singh Khalsa (Yogi Bhajan). Class Lecture. <u>Breaking Through the Mask</u>. 15 Nov 1983. Meditation information can be retrieved from
        <https://docs.google.com/viewer?url=http://www.ikyta.org/clients/ikyta/webshell.nsf/0/59f66d297abaeab3872572bc0004b10f/$FILE/KR_Spring_08.pdf>

[78] Ibid

[79] Raj Karega Khalsa Network. <u>Basant Ki Vaar</u>. Retrieved 12 Feb 2011 from
        <http://www.rajkaregakhalsa.net/basant_ki_vaar.htm>

[80] Yogi Bhajan, Ph.D., (2003) *The Aquarian Teacher: KRI International Kundalini Yoga Teacher Training Level I.* (p. 85). Kundalini Research Institute.

[81] SSS Harbhajan Singh Khalsa (Yogi Bhajan). Class Lecture. <u>Experience Your Own Soul Blessing You with Prosperity</u>. Meditation information can be retrieved from
        <http://www.dasvandh.org/meditations/experience-your-own-soul-blessing-you-prosperity>

[82] Yogi Bhajan, Ph.D., (2003) *The Aquarian Teacher: KRI International Kundalini Yoga Teacher Training Level I.* (p. 433). Kundalini Research Institute.

[83] Yogi Bhajan, Ph.D., (2003) *The Aquarian Teacher: KRI International Kundalini Yoga Teacher Training Level I.* (p. 423). Kundalini Research Institute.

[84] Yogi Bhajan, Ph.D., (2003) *The Aquarian Teacher: KRI International Kundalini Yoga Teacher Training Level I.* (p. 85). Kundalini Research Institute.

[85] Spirit Voyage Music. <u>Mantra-Pedia: Jai Te Gang</u>. Retrieved on 10 February 2011 from
        <http://www.spiritvoyage.com/mantra/Jai-Te-Gang/MAN-000119.aspx>

[86] SSS Harbhajan Singh Khalsa (Yogi Bhajan). Class Lecture. <u>Jei Te Gang</u>. 07 May 1989.

[87] SSS Harbhajan Singh Khalsa (Yogi Bhajan). Class Lecture. 01 Oct 1989.

[88] Translation adapted from: *Nit Naym*. (1987) . Handmade Books.

[89] SSS Harbhajan Singh Khalsa (Yogi Bhajan). Class Lecture. <u>Kauri Kriya</u>. Española, 1976. Class notes originally taken by and appear courtesy of Sat Kirin Kaur Khalsa. Complete class notes are available at www.thedivineportal.com upon request.

[90] Ibid

[91] Ibid

[92] Yogi Bhajan, Ph.D., (2003) *The Aquarian Teacher: KRI International Kundalini Yoga Teacher Training Level I.* (p. 418). Kundalini Research Institute.

[93] Ibid

[94] Yogi Bhajan, Ph.D., (2001) *Meditations for the New Millennium.* (#LA0963). Kundalini Research Institute. Originally taught in Los Angeles, 03 March 2001.

[95] Translation adapted from: <u>The Shiva Prayer Book</u>. Retrieved on 12 Feb 2011 from
        <http://www.vishuji.org/shivpuja.htm>

[96] Word for word translations provided by: Nandhi. <u>Maha Mrityunjaya Mantra</u>. Retrieved on 12 Feb 2011 from
        <http://www.nandhi.com/mrityunjaya.htm>

[97] Gannon, Sharonji. Class Notes. <u>Maha Mrityunjai Mantra</u>. Omega Institute. May 2007.

[98] Translation adapted from: Raj Karega Khalsa Network. <u>Mangal Saaj Ba-i-aa</u>. Retrieved 12 Feb 2011 from
        <http://www.rajkaregakhalsa.net/Gurbani/Amrit_Kirtan/tr_1059.html>

[99] Khalsa, Siri Kirpal Kaur, (2002) *Yoga for Prosperity*. (p.50). Santa Cruz, NM, USA: Yogiji Press

[100] Yogi Bhajan, Ph.D., <u>Meditation to Heal the Wounds of Love</u>. Retrieved on 12 Feb 2011 from
        <http://www.3ho.org/kundalini-yoga/kundalini-yoga-yb/kriyas-meditations/featured-meditations/pdfs/MeditateHealWoundsLove.pdf>

[101] Translation adapted from: Sikhnet. <u>Healing The Wounds Of Love By Guru Raj Kaur And Nirinjan Kaur</u>. Retrieved on 12 Feb 2011 from
        < http://www.sikhnet.com/content/healing-wounds-love-guru-raj-kaur-and-nirinjan-kaur >

[102] SSS Harbhajan Singh Khalsa (Yogi Bhajan). Class Lecture. <u>An Attitude of Deathlessness</u>. 12 March 1989. Transcript by Tej Kaur. Los Angeles, CA.

[103] Lyrics appear with permission of Livtar Singh

[104] Khalsa, Harijot Kaur, and Yogi Bhajan, Ph.D., (2006) *Praana Praanee Praanayam Exploring the Breath Technology of Kundalini Yoga as Taught by Yogi Bhajan®.* (p. 35-6). Española, NM, USA: Kundalini Research Institute.

[105] Yogi Bhajan, Ph.D., (2003) *The Aquarian Teacher: KRI International Kundalini Yoga Teacher Training Level I.* (p. 86). Kundalini Research Institute.

[106] Yogi Bhajan, Ph.D., (2003) *The Aquarian Teacher: KRI International Kundalini Yoga Teacher Training Level I.* (p. 447). Kundalini Research Institute.

[107] Ibid

[108] Kaur, Snatam. "People of Love". <u>Celebrate Peace</u>. Spirit Voyage Music, 2005. CD. Lyrics appear with permission from Snatam Kaur.

[109] Yogi Bhajan, Ph.D., (2003) *The Aquarian Teacher: KRI International Kundalini Yoga Teacher Training Level I.* (p. 174). Kundalini Research Institute.

[110] Swami Muktibodhananda, (2005) *Hatha Yoga Pradipika.* (p.619). Bihar, India: Yoga Publications Trust.

[111] Yogi Bhajan, Ph.D., (2003) *The Aquarian Teacher: KRI International Kundalini Yoga Teacher Training Level I.* (p. 422). Kundalini Research Institute.

[112] Khalasa, Shakti Parwa Kaur, (1996) *Kundalini Yoga: The Flow of Eternal Power.* (Meditation to Develop Effective Communication p.214). New York: The Berkeley Publishing Group.

[113] *Mantras in Motion.* Gurudass Kaur. 2007. DVD.

[114] SSS Harbhajan Singh Khalsa (Yogi Bhajan). <u>Mantra-Pedia: Ram Ram Hari Ram</u>. Retrieved on 12 Feb 2011 from

<http://www.spiritvoyage.com/mantra/Ram-Ram-Hari-Ram/MAN-000114.aspx>

[115] Ibid

[116] Translation by Snatam Kaur. Retrieved on 13 Feb 2011 from
<http://www.snatamkaur.com/web7.html >

[117] Khalsa, Mahan Kirn Kaur, (2005) *Bound Lotus: An Instructional Manual.* (p.51). USA: Spirit Voyage Publishing (ASCAP).

[118] Yogi Bhajan, Ph.D., (2003) *The Aquarian Teacher: KRI International Kundalini Yoga Teacher Training Level I. (*p. 412).
Kundalini Research Institute.

[119] SSS Harbhajan Singh Khalsa (Yogi Bhajan). Mantra-Pedia: Sat Kartar. Retrieved on 13 Feb 2011 from
<http://www.spiritvoyage.com/mantra/Sat-Kartar/MAN-000104.aspx>

[120] Ibid

[121] SSS Harbhajan Singh Khalsa (Yogi Bhajan). (2010). Fire Kriya. Originally taught on 20 March 1978. Retrieved on 13 Feb 2011
from
<https://docs.google.com/viewer?url=http://www.3ho.org/get-involved/images/firekriya2010.pdf>

[122] Ibid

[123] Yogi Bhajan, Ph.D. and Gurucharan Singh Khalsa Ph.D., (1998) *The Mind: Its Projections and Multiple Facets.. (*p. 170).
Kundalini Research Institute.

[124] SSS Harbhajan Singh Khalsa (Yogi Bhajan). (2009). 2009 Meditation: The Water Element – Narayan Kriya – Clearing and Clarity
for Prosperity. Retrieved on 13 Feb 2011 from
<https://docs.google.com/viewer?url=http://www.3ho.org/kundalini-yoga/kundalini-yoga-yb/kriyas-meditations/featured-
meditations/pdfs/2009NarayanKriya.pdf>

[125] Kaur, Sat Avtar. Kundalini Yoga Mantras Starting with S: Sat Narayan. (2011). Retrieved on 13 Feb 2011 from
<http://www.kundalini-yoga-info.com/sarega.html#satnarchotay>

[126] Khalsa Md., Singh Sahib Sant. Gurmukhi to English Translation and Phonetic Transliteration of Siri Guru Granth Sahib: Sentence
by Sentence. (p. 10). Retrieved on 13 Feb 2011 from
<http://www.sikhnet.com/oldsikhnet/sggs/translation/0010.html>
Translation appears with Permission from Singh Sahib Sant Khalsa Md.

[127] Spirit Voyage Music. Paraphrasing the teachings of SSS Harbhajan Singh Khalsa (Yogi Bhajan). Mantra-Pedia: So Purkh.
Retrieved on 13 Feb 2011 from
< http://www.spiritvoyage.com/mantra/So-Purkh/MAN-000107.aspx>

[128] Spirit Voyage Music. Mantra-pedia: Teree Meher Daa Bolnaa. Retrieved on 13 Feb 2011 from
<http://www.spiritvoyage.com/mantra/Teree-Meher-Daa-Bolnaa/MAN-000108.aspx>

[129] Kaur, Snatam. Mantra-pedia: Teree Meher Daa Bolnaa. Retrieved on 13 Feb 2011 from
<http://www.spiritvoyage.com/mantra/Teree-Meher-Daa-Bolnaa/MAN-000108.aspx>

[130] SSS Harbhajan Singh Khalsa (Yogi Bhajan). (Jan 2008). 3HO enewsletter – A Meditation for 2008 from Gurucharan Singh.
Retrieved on 14 Feb 2011 from
<http://www.3ho.org/enewsletter/e-news01-01-08.html>

[131] Ibid

[132] Spirit Voyage Music. Mantra-pedia: Triple Mantra. Retrieved on 13 Feb 2011 from
<http://www.spiritvoyage.com/mantra/Triple-Mantra/MAN-000109.aspx>

[133] SSS Harbhajan Singh Khalsa (Yogi Bhajan). (2012). Air Tattva: The 2012 Global Meditation. Retrieved on 14 Mar
2014 from
<http://www.3ho.org/kundalini-yoga/mantra/2012-ether-tattva-mantra>

[134] SSS Harbhajan Singh Khalsa (Yogi Bhajan). Class Lecture. The Keystone of Prosperity. 24 Sept 1989. Transcript by Tej Kaur.
Los Angeles, CA.

[135] Yogi Bhajan, Ph.D. and Gurucharan Singh Khalsa Ph.D., (1998) *The Mind: Its Projections and Multiple Facets.. (*p. 175).
Kundalini Research Institute.

[136] Ibid

[137] Kaur, Snatam. "We Are Peace". Celebrate Peace. Spirit Voyage Music, 2005. CD. Lyrics appear with permission from Snatam
Kaur.

[138] The Sikh Encyclopedia. Nitnem: Posted in Philosophy, Spirituality and Ethics – Moral Codes and Sikh Practices. Retrieved on 14
Feb 2011 from
<http://www.thesikhencyclopedia.com/moral-codes-and-sikh-practices/nitnem.html>

[139] SSS Harbhajan Singh Khalsa (Yogi Bhajan). Class Lecture. The Sikh Gurus. 01 Oct 1987. Transcript by Tej Kaur. Los Angeles,
CA.

[140] Chhath Puja. Guru Nanak Jayanti. Retrieved on 14 Feb 2011 from
<http://www.chhathpuja.co/community/groups/viewbulletin/125-Guru+Nanak+Jayanti?groupid=86>

[141] Paraphrased from class lecture given by Gurushabd Singh Khalsa at The Omega Institute for Holistic Studies. Oct 2004.
Rhinebeck, NY. Along with excerts from: Yogi Bhajan, Ph.D., (2003) *The Aquarian Teacher: KRI International Kundalini
Yoga Teacher Training Level I. (*p. 81). Kundalini Research Institute.

[142] Yogi Bhajan, Ph.D., (2003) *The Aquarian Teacher: KRI International Kundalini Yoga Teacher Training Level I. (*p. 80). Kundalini
Research Institute.

[143] Translation adapted from the following: Harbans Singh Doabia (2005), *Sacred Nitnem* (26th ed.). (p. 249) Amritsar, India: Singh
Brothers Publishers. Translation appears with Permission from Singh Brothers Publishers and Khalsa Md., Singh Sahib
Sant. Gurmukhi to English Translation and Phonetic Transliteration of Siri Guru Granth Sahib: Sentence by Sentence. (p. 1).
Retrieved on 16 Feb 2011 from
< http://www.sikhnet.com/oldsikhnet/sggs/translation/0001.html>
Translation appears with Permission from Singh Sahib Sant Khalsa Md.

[144] Yogi Bhajan, Ph.D., (2003) *The Aquarian Teacher: KRI International Kundalini Yoga Teacher Training Level I.* (p. 80). Kundalini Research Institute.

[145] Translation adapted from the following: Harbans Singh Doabia (2005), *Sacred Nitnem* (26th ed.). (p. 249) Amritsar, India: Singh Brothers Publishers. Translation appears with Permission from Singh Brothers Publishers and Khalsa Md., Singh Sahib Sant. Gurmukhi to English Translation and Phonetic Transliteration of Siri Guru Granth Sahib: Sentence by Sentence. (p. 1). Retrieved on 16 Feb 2011 from
< http://www.sikhnet.com/oldsikhnet/sggs/translation/0001.html>
Translation appears with Permission from Singh Sahib Sant Khalsa Md.

[146] Khalsa, Guruliv Singh. "Guru Arjun's Love Letters". Stories For Khalsa Children. Invincible Recordings. CD

[147] Yogi Bhajan, Ph.D., Meditation to Heal the Wounds of Love. Retrieved on 12 Feb 2011 from
<http://www.3ho.org/kundalini-yoga/kundalini-yoga-yb/kriyas-meditations/featured-meditations/pdfs/MeditateHealWoundsLove.pdf>

[148] SSS Harbhajan Singh Khalsa (Yogi Bhajan). Class Lecture. The Law of Life. 01 July 1987.

[149] Khalsa Md., Singh Sahib Sant. Shabad Hazaray – Eng – Rom - Gurm. Retrieved on 18 Feb 2011 from
<https://docs.google.com/viewer?url=http://www.sikhnet.com/sikhnet/Register.nsf/Files/PDABanis/$file/Shabad%2520Hazaray%2520-%2520Eng-Rom-Gurm.doc>
Translation appears with Permission from Singh Sahib Sant Khalsa Md.

[150] SSS Harbhajan Singh Khalsa (Yogi Bhajan). (1983). *Kundalini Yoga for Youth & Joy*. (p.58). Eugene: 3HO Transcripts.

[151] Harbans Singh Doabia (2005), *Sacred Nitnem* (26th ed.). (p. 72 - 143) Amritsar, India: Singh Brothers Publishers. Translation appears with Permission from Singh Brothers Publishers.

[152] Translation adapted from: Harbans Singh Doabia (2005), *Sacred Nitnem* (26th ed.). (p. 146 - 155) Amritsar, India: Singh Brothers Publishers. Translation appears with Permission from Singh Brothers Publishers.

[153] Khalsa, Guruliv Singh. "Creation of Anand Sahib". Stories For Khalsa Children. Invincible Recordings. CD

[154] Translation of first stanza from: Anand Sahib. (09 May 2010). Retrieved on 10 Feb 2011 from
<http://www.sikhiwiki.org/index.php/Anand_sahib>

[155] Translation of remainder of Anand Sahib from: Khalsa Md., Singh Sahib Sant. Anand Sahib – Eng-Translation. Retrieved on 22 Feb 2011 from
<https://docs.google.com/viewer?url=http://fateh.sikhnet.com/sikhnet/Register.nsf/Files/PDABanis/$file/Anand%2520Sahib%2520-%2520Eng-Translation.doc>
Translation appears with Permission from Singh Sahib Sant Khalsa Md.

[156] Rehiras Sahib. Retrieved on 28 Feb 2011 from
<http://www.sikhphilosophy.net/gurmat-vichaar/17342-rehiras-sahib-sampooran-sikh-prayer.html>

[157] Translation adapted from: Harbans Singh Doabia (2005), *Sacred Nitnem* (26th ed.). (p. 204 - 249) Amritsar, India: Singh Brothers Publishers. Translation appears with Permission from Singh Brothers Publishers. Translation also adapted from: Rehiras. Retrieved on 28 Feb 2011 from
<http://www.rajkaregakhalsa.net/RehirasSahibji.htm>

[158] Kirtan Sohila. Retrieved on 28 Feb 2011 from
< http://www.sikhiwiki.org/index.php/Kirtan_Sohila>

[159] Harbans Singh Doabia (2005), *Sacred Nitnem* (26th ed.). (p. 263) Amritsar, India: Singh Brothers Publishers. Translation appears with Permission from Singh Brothers Publishers.

[160] Khalsa Md., Singh Sahib Sant. Gurmukhi to English Translation and Phonetic Transliteration of Siri Guru Granth Sahib: Sentence by Sentence. (p. 12). Retrieved on 28 Feb 2011 from
<http://www.sikhnet.com/oldsikhnet/sggs/translation/0012.html>
Translation appears with Permission from Singh Sahib Sant Khalsa Md.

INDEX

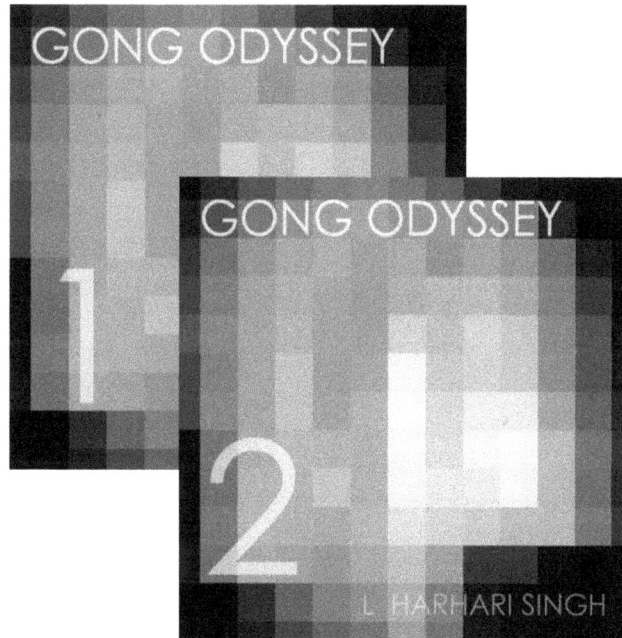

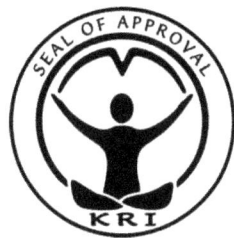

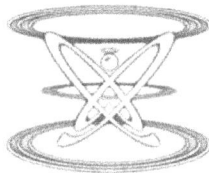

WWW.THEDIVINEPORTAL.COM

www.ingramcontent.com/pod-product-compliance
Lightning Source LLC
Chambersburg PA
CBHW062044090426
42740CB00016B/3011